FREE Study Skills Videos/

Dear Customer,

Thank you for your purchase from Mometrix! We consider it an honor and a privilege that you have purchased our product and we want to ensure your satisfaction.

As part of our ongoing effort to meet the needs of test takers, we have developed a set of Study Skills Videos that we would like to give you for <u>FREE</u>. These videos cover our *best practices* for getting ready for your exam, from how to use our study materials to how to best prepare for the day of the test.

All that we ask is that you email us with feedback that would describe your experience so far with our product. Good, bad, or indifferent, we want to know what you think!

To get your FREE Study Skills Videos, you can use the **QR code** below, or send us an **email** at studyvideos@mometrix.com with *FREE VIDEOS* in the subject line and the following information in the body of the email:

- The name of the product you purchased.
- Your product rating on a scale of 1-5, with 5 being the highest rating.
- Your feedback. It can be long, short, or anything in between. We just want to know your impressions and experience so far with our product. (Good feedback might include how our study material met your needs and ways we might be able to make it even better. You could highlight features that you found helpful or features that you think we should add.)

If you have any questions or concerns, please don't hesitate to contact me directly.

Thanks again!

Sincerely,

Jay Willis
Vice President
jay.willis@mometrix.com
1-800-673-8175

SCAN HERE

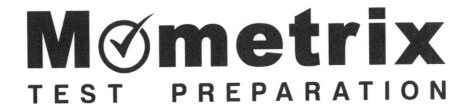

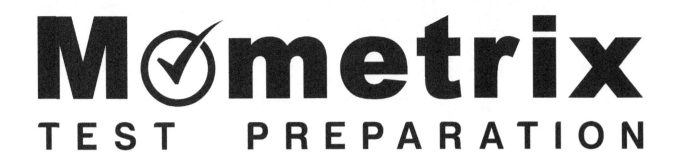

NHA Phlebotomy

Exam Prep 2023-2024

4 Full-Length Practice Tests

Secrets Study Guide Book for the NHA Certification

3rd Edition

Written and edited by Mometrix Test Prep

Printed in the United States of America

This paper meets the requirements of ANSI/NISO Z39.48-1992 (Permanence of Paper).

Mometrix offers volume discount pricing to institutions. For more information or a price quote, please contact our sales department at sales@mometrix.com or 888-248-1219.

Mometrix Media LLC is not affiliated with or endorsed by any official testing organization. All organizational and test names are trademarks of their respective owners.

Paperback
ISBN 13: 978-1-5167-2403-1
ISBN 10: 1-5167-2403-8

DEAR FUTURE EXAM SUCCESS STORY

First of all, **THANK YOU** for purchasing Mometrix study materials!

Second, congratulations! You are one of the few determined test-takers who are committed to doing whatever it takes to excel on your exam. **You have come to the right place.** We developed these study materials with one goal in mind: to deliver you the information you need in a format that's concise and easy to use.

In addition to optimizing your guide for the content of the test, we've outlined our recommended steps for breaking down the preparation process into small, attainable goals so you can make sure you stay on track.

We've also analyzed the entire test-taking process, identifying the most common pitfalls and showing how you can overcome them and be ready for any curveball the test throws you.

Standardized testing is one of the biggest obstacles on your road to success, which only increases the importance of doing well in the high-pressure, high-stakes environment of test day. Your results on this test could have a significant impact on your future, and this guide provides the information and practical advice to help you achieve your full potential on test day.

Your success is our success

We would love to hear from you! If you would like to share the story of your exam success or if you have any questions or comments in regard to our products, please contact us at **800-673-8175** or **support@mometrix.com**.

Thanks again for your business and we wish you continued success!

Sincerely,
The Mometrix Test Preparation Team

> **Need more help? Check out our flashcards at:**
> **http://MometrixFlashcards.com/Phlebotomy**

TABLE OF CONTENTS

Introduction

Thank you for purchasing this resource! You have made the choice to prepare yourself for a test that could have a huge impact on your future, and this guide is designed to help you be fully ready for test day. Obviously, it's important to have a solid understanding of the test material, but you also need to be prepared for the unique environment and stressors of the test, so that you can perform to the best of your abilities.

For this purpose, the first section that appears in this guide is the **Secret Keys**. We've devoted countless hours to meticulously researching what works and what doesn't, and we've boiled down our findings to the five most impactful steps you can take to improve your performance on the test. We start at the beginning with study planning and move through the preparation process, all the way to the testing strategies that will help you get the most out of what you know when you're finally sitting in front of the test.

We recommend that you start preparing for your test as far in advance as possible. However, if you've bought this guide as a last-minute study resource and only have a few days before your test, we recommend that you skip over the first two Secret Keys since they address a long-term study plan.

If you struggle with **test anxiety**, we strongly encourage you to check out our recommendations for how you can overcome it. Test anxiety is a formidable foe, but it can be beaten, and we want to make sure you have the tools you need to defeat it.

1

Secret Key #1 – Plan Big, Study Small

There's a lot riding on your performance. If you want to ace this test, you're going to need to keep your skills sharp and the material fresh in your mind. You need a plan that lets you review everything you need to know while still fitting in your schedule. We'll break this strategy down into three categories.

Information Organization

Start with the information you already have: the official test outline. From this, you can make a complete list of all the concepts you need to cover before the test. Organize these concepts into groups that can be studied together, and create a list of any related vocabulary you need to learn so you can brush up on any difficult terms. You'll want to keep this vocabulary list handy once you actually start studying since you may need to add to it along the way.

Time Management

Once you have your set of study concepts, decide how to spread them out over the time you have left before the test. Break your study plan into small, clear goals so you have a manageable task for each day and know exactly what you're doing. Then just focus on one small step at a time. When you manage your time this way, you don't need to spend hours at a time studying. Studying a small block of content for a short period each day helps you retain information better and avoid stressing over how much you have left to do. You can relax knowing that you have a plan to cover everything in time. In order for this strategy to be effective though, you have to start studying early and stick to your schedule. Avoid the exhaustion and futility that comes from last-minute cramming!

Study Environment

The environment you study in has a big impact on your learning. Studying in a coffee shop, while probably more enjoyable, is not likely to be as fruitful as studying in a quiet room. It's important to keep distractions to a minimum. You're only planning to study for a short block of time, so make the most of it. Don't pause to check your phone or get up to find a snack. It's also important to **avoid multitasking**. Research has consistently shown that multitasking will make your studying dramatically less effective. Your study area should also be comfortable and well-lit so you don't have the distraction of straining your eyes or sitting on an uncomfortable chair.

 The time of day you study is also important. You want to be rested and alert. Don't wait until just before bedtime. Study when you'll be most likely to comprehend and remember. Even better, if you know what time of day your test will be, set that time aside for study. That way your brain will be used to working on that subject at that specific time and you'll have a better chance of recalling information.

Finally, it can be helpful to team up with others who are studying for the same test. Your actual studying should be done in as isolated an environment as possible, but the work of organizing the information and setting up the study plan can be divided up. In between study sessions, you can discuss with your teammates the concepts that you're all studying and quiz each other on the details. Just be sure that your teammates are as serious about the test as you are. If you find that your study time is being replaced with social time, you might need to find a new team.

Secret Key #2 – Make Your Studying Count

You're devoting a lot of time and effort to preparing for this test, so you want to be absolutely certain it will pay off. This means doing more than just reading the content and hoping you can remember it on test day. It's important to make every minute of study count. There are two main areas you can focus on to make your studying count.

Retention

It doesn't matter how much time you study if you can't remember the material. You need to make sure you are retaining the concepts. To check your retention of the information you're learning, try recalling it at later times with minimal prompting. Try carrying around flashcards and glance at one or two from time to time or ask a friend who's also studying for the test to quiz you.

To enhance your retention, look for ways to put the information into practice so that you can apply it rather than simply recalling it. If you're using the information in practical ways, it will be much easier to remember. Similarly, it helps to solidify a concept in your mind if you're not only reading it to yourself but also explaining it to someone else. Ask a friend to let you teach them about a concept you're a little shaky on (or speak aloud to an imaginary audience if necessary). As you try to summarize, define, give examples, and answer your friend's questions, you'll understand the concepts better and they will stay with you longer. Finally, step back for a big picture view and ask yourself how each piece of information fits with the whole subject. When you link the different concepts together and see them working together as a whole, it's easier to remember the individual components.

Finally, practice showing your work on any multi-step problems, even if you're just studying. Writing out each step you take to solve a problem will help solidify the process in your mind, and you'll be more likely to remember it during the test.

Modality

Modality simply refers to the means or method by which you study. Choosing a study modality that fits your own individual learning style is crucial. No two people learn best in exactly the same way, so it's important to know your strengths and use them to your advantage.

For example, if you learn best by visualization, focus on visualizing a concept in your mind and draw an image or a diagram. Try color-coding your notes, illustrating them, or creating symbols that will trigger your mind to recall a learned concept. If you learn best by hearing or discussing information, find a study partner who learns the same way or read aloud to yourself. Think about how to put the information in your own words. Imagine that you are giving a lecture on the topic and record yourself so you can listen to it later.

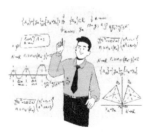

For any learning style, flashcards can be helpful. Organize the information so you can take advantage of spare moments to review. Underline key words or phrases. Use different colors for different categories. Mnemonic devices (such as creating a short list in which every item starts with the same letter) can also help with retention. Find what works best for you and use it to store the information in your mind most effectively and easily.

3

Secret Key #3 – Practice the Right Way

Your success on test day depends not only on how many hours you put into preparing, but also on whether you prepared the right way. It's good to check along the way to see if your studying is paying off. One of the most effective ways to do this is by taking practice tests to evaluate your progress. Practice tests are useful because they show exactly where you need to improve. Every time you take a practice test, pay special attention to these three groups of questions:

- The questions you got wrong
- The questions you had to guess on, even if you guessed right
- The questions you found difficult or slow to work through

This will show you exactly what your weak areas are, and where you need to devote more study time. Ask yourself why each of these questions gave you trouble. Was it because you didn't understand the material? Was it because you didn't remember the vocabulary? Do you need more repetitions on this type of question to build speed and confidence? Dig into those questions and figure out how you can strengthen your weak areas as you go back to review the material.

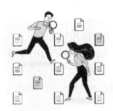 Additionally, many practice tests have a section explaining the answer choices. It can be tempting to read the explanation and think that you now have a good understanding of the concept. However, an explanation likely only covers part of the question's broader context. Even if the explanation makes perfect sense, **go back and investigate** every concept related to the question until you're positive you have a thorough understanding.

As you go along, keep in mind that the practice test is just that: practice. Memorizing these questions and answers will not be very helpful on the actual test because it is unlikely to have any of the same exact questions. If you only know the right answers to the sample questions, you won't be prepared for the real thing. **Study the concepts** until you understand them fully, and then you'll be able to answer any question that shows up on the test.

It's important to wait on the practice tests until you're ready. If you take a test on your first day of study, you may be overwhelmed by the amount of material covered and how much you need to learn. Work up to it gradually.

On test day, you'll need to be prepared for answering questions, managing your time, and using the test-taking strategies you've learned. It's a lot to balance, like a mental marathon that will have a big impact on your future. Like training for a marathon, you'll need to start slowly and work your way up. When test day arrives, you'll be ready.

Start with the strategies you've read in the first two Secret Keys—plan your course and study in the way that works best for you. If you have time, consider using multiple study resources to get different approaches to the same concepts. It can be helpful to see difficult concepts from more than one angle. Then find a good source for practice tests. Many times, the test website will suggest potential study resources or provide sample tests.

4

Practice Test Strategy

If you're able to find at least three practice tests, we recommend this strategy:

UNTIMED AND OPEN-BOOK PRACTICE

Take the first test with no time constraints and with your notes and study guide handy. Take your time and focus on applying the strategies you've learned.

TIMED AND OPEN-BOOK PRACTICE

Take the second practice test open-book as well, but set a timer and practice pacing yourself to finish in time.

TIMED AND CLOSED-BOOK PRACTICE

Take any other practice tests as if it were test day. Set a timer and put away your study materials. Sit at a table or desk in a quiet room, imagine yourself at the testing center, and answer questions as quickly and accurately as possible.

Keep repeating timed and closed-book tests on a regular basis until you run out of practice tests or it's time for the actual test. Your mind will be ready for the schedule and stress of test day, and you'll be able to focus on recalling the material you've learned.

Secret Key #4 – Pace Yourself

Once you're fully prepared for the material on the test, your biggest challenge on test day will be managing your time. Just knowing that the clock is ticking can make you panic even if you have plenty of time left. Work on pacing yourself so you can build confidence against the time constraints of the exam. Pacing is a difficult skill to master, especially in a high-pressure environment, so **practice is vital**.

Set time expectations for your pace based on how much time is available. For example, if a section has 60 questions and the time limit is 30 minutes, you know you have to average 30 seconds or less per question in order to answer them all. Although 30 seconds is the hard limit, set 25 seconds per question as your goal, so you reserve extra time to spend on harder questions. When you budget extra time for the harder questions, you no longer have any reason to stress when those questions take longer to answer.

Don't let this time expectation distract you from working through the test at a calm, steady pace, but keep it in mind so you don't spend too much time on any one question. Recognize that taking extra time on one question you don't understand may keep you from answering two that you do understand later in the test. If your time limit for a question is up and you're still not sure of the answer, mark it and move on, and come back to it later if the time and the test format allow. If the testing format doesn't allow you to return to earlier questions, just make an educated guess; then put it out of your mind and move on.

On the easier questions, be careful not to rush. It may seem wise to hurry through them so you have more time for the challenging ones, but it's not worth missing one if you know the concept and just didn't take the time to read the question fully. Work efficiently but make sure you understand the question and have looked at all of the answer choices, since more than one may seem right at first.

Even if you're paying attention to the time, you may find yourself a little behind at some point. You should speed up to get back on track, but do so wisely. Don't panic; just take a few seconds less on each question until you're caught up. Don't guess without thinking, but do look through the answer choices and eliminate any you know are wrong. If you can get down to two choices, it is often worthwhile to guess from those. Once you've chosen an answer, move on and don't dwell on any that you skipped or had to hurry through. If a question was taking too long, chances are it was one of the harder ones, so you weren't as likely to get it right anyway.

On the other hand, if you find yourself getting ahead of schedule, it may be beneficial to slow down a little. The more quickly you work, the more likely you are to make a careless mistake that will affect your score. You've budgeted time for each question, so don't be afraid to spend that time. Practice an efficient but careful pace to get the most out of the time you have.

Secret Key #5 – Have a Plan for Guessing

When you're taking the test, you may find yourself stuck on a question. Some of the answer choices seem better than others, but you don't see the one answer choice that is obviously correct. What do you do?

The scenario described above is very common, yet most test takers have not effectively prepared for it. Developing and practicing a plan for guessing may be one of the single most effective uses of your time as you get ready for the exam.

In developing your plan for guessing, there are three questions to address:

- When should you start the guessing process?
- How should you narrow down the choices?
- Which answer should you choose?

When to Start the Guessing Process

Unless your plan for guessing is to select C every time (which, despite its merits, is not what we recommend), you need to leave yourself enough time to apply your answer elimination strategies. Since you have a limited amount of time for each question, that means that if you're going to give yourself the best shot at guessing correctly, you have to decide quickly whether or not you will guess.

Of course, the best-case scenario is that you don't have to guess at all, so first, see if you can answer the question based on your knowledge of the subject and basic reasoning skills. Focus on the key words in the question and try to jog your memory of related topics. Give yourself a chance to bring the knowledge to mind, but once you realize that you don't have (or you can't access) the knowledge you need to answer the question, it's time to start the guessing process.

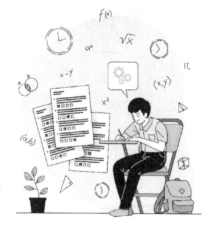

It's almost always better to start the guessing process too early than too late. It only takes a few seconds to remember something and answer the question from knowledge. Carefully eliminating wrong answer choices takes longer. Plus, going through the process of eliminating answer choices can actually help jog your memory.

Summary: Start the guessing process as soon as you decide that you can't answer the question based on your knowledge.

7

How to Narrow Down the Choices

The next chapter in this book (**Test-Taking Strategies**) includes a wide range of strategies for how to approach questions and how to look for answer choices to eliminate. You will definitely want to read those carefully, practice them, and figure out which ones work best for you. Here though, we're going to address a mindset rather than a particular strategy.

Your odds of guessing an answer correctly depend on how many options you are choosing from.

Number of options left	5	4	3	2	1
Odds of guessing correctly	20%	25%	33%	50%	100%

You can see from this chart just how valuable it is to be able to eliminate incorrect answers and make an educated guess, but there are two things that many test takers do that cause them to miss out on the benefits of guessing:

- Accidentally eliminating the correct answer
- Selecting an answer based on an impression

We'll look at the first one here, and the second one in the next section.

To avoid accidentally eliminating the correct answer, we recommend a thought exercise called **the $5 challenge**. In this challenge, you only eliminate an answer choice from contention if you are willing to bet $5 on it being wrong. Why $5? Five dollars is a small but not insignificant amount of money. It's an amount you could afford to lose but wouldn't want to throw away. And while losing

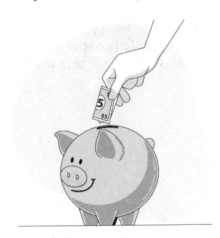

$5 once might not hurt too much, doing it twenty times will set you back $100. In the same way, each small decision you make—eliminating a choice here, guessing on a question there—won't by itself impact your score very much, but when you put them all together, they can make a big difference. By holding each answer choice elimination decision to a higher standard, you can reduce the risk of accidentally eliminating the correct answer.

The $5 challenge can also be applied in a positive sense: If you are willing to bet $5 that an answer choice *is* correct, go ahead and mark it as correct.

Summary: Only eliminate an answer choice if you are willing to bet $5 that it is wrong.

8

Which Answer to Choose

You're taking the test. You've run into a hard question and decided you'll have to guess. You've eliminated all the answer choices you're willing to bet $5 on. Now you have to pick an answer. Why do we even need to talk about this? Why can't you just pick whichever one you feel like when the time comes?

The answer to these questions is that if you don't come into the test with a plan, you'll rely on your impression to select an answer choice, and if you do that, you risk falling into a trap. The test writers know that everyone who takes their test will be guessing on some of the questions, so they intentionally write wrong answer choices to seem plausible. You still have to pick an answer though, and if the wrong answer choices are designed to look right, how can you ever be sure that you're not falling for their trap? The best solution we've found to this dilemma is to take the decision out of your hands entirely. Here is the process we recommend:

Once you've eliminated any choices that you are confident (willing to bet $5) are wrong, select the first remaining choice as your answer.

Whether you choose to select the first remaining choice, the second, or the last, the important thing is that you use some preselected standard. Using this approach guarantees that you will not be enticed into selecting an answer choice that looks right, because you are not basing your decision on how the answer choices look.

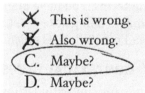

This is not meant to make you question your knowledge. Instead, it is to help you recognize the difference between your knowledge and your impressions. There's a huge difference between thinking an answer is right because of what you know, and thinking an answer is right because it looks or sounds like it should be right.

Summary: To ensure that your selection is appropriately random, make a predetermined selection from among all answer choices you have not eliminated.

Test-Taking Strategies

This section contains a list of test-taking strategies that you may find helpful as you work through the test. By taking what you know and applying logical thought, you can maximize your chances of answering any question correctly!

It is very important to realize that every question is different and every person is different: no single strategy will work on every question, and no single strategy will work for every person. That's why we've included all of them here, so you can try them out and determine which ones work best for different types of questions and which ones work best for you.

Question Strategies

☑ READ CAREFULLY

Read the question and the answer choices carefully. Don't miss the question because you misread the terms. You have plenty of time to read each question thoroughly and make sure you understand what is being asked. Yet a happy medium must be attained, so don't waste too much time. You must read carefully and efficiently.

☑ CONTEXTUAL CLUES

Look for contextual clues. If the question includes a word you are not familiar with, look at the immediate context for some indication of what the word might mean. Contextual clues can often give you all the information you need to decipher the meaning of an unfamiliar word. Even if you can't determine the meaning, you may be able to narrow down the possibilities enough to make a solid guess at the answer to the question.

☑ PREFIXES

If you're having trouble with a word in the question or answer choices, try dissecting it. Take advantage of every clue that the word might include. Prefixes can be a huge help. Usually, they allow you to determine a basic meaning. *Pre-* means before, *post-* means after, *pro-* is positive, *de-* is negative. From prefixes, you can get an idea of the general meaning of the word and try to put it into context.

☑ HEDGE WORDS

Watch out for critical hedge words, such as *likely, may, can, sometimes, often, almost, mostly, usually, generally, rarely,* and *sometimes*. Question writers insert these hedge phrases to cover every possibility. Often an answer choice will be wrong simply because it leaves no room for exception. Be on guard for answer choices that have definitive words such as *exactly* and *always*.

☑ SWITCHBACK WORDS

Stay alert for *switchbacks*. These are the words and phrases frequently used to alert you to shifts in thought. The most common switchback words are *but, although,* and *however*. Others include *nevertheless, on the other hand, even though, while, in spite of, despite,* and *regardless of*. Switchback words are important to catch because they can change the direction of the question or an answer choice.

⊘ Face Value

When in doubt, use common sense. Accept the situation in the problem at face value. Don't read too much into it. These problems will not require you to make wild assumptions. If you have to go beyond creativity and warp time or space in order to have an answer choice fit the question, then you should move on and consider the other answer choices. These are normal problems rooted in reality. The applicable relationship or explanation may not be readily apparent, but it is there for you to figure out. Use your common sense to interpret anything that isn't clear.

Answer Choice Strategies

⊘ Answer Selection

The most thorough way to pick an answer choice is to identify and eliminate wrong answers until only one is left, then confirm it is the correct answer. Sometimes an answer choice may immediately seem right, but be careful. The test writers will usually put more than one reasonable answer choice on each question, so take a second to read all of them and make sure that the other choices are not equally obvious. As long as you have time left, it is better to read every answer choice than to pick the first one that looks right without checking the others.

⊘ Answer Choice Families

An answer choice family consists of two (in rare cases, three) answer choices that are very similar in construction and cannot all be true at the same time. If you see two answer choices that are direct opposites or parallels, one of them is usually the correct answer. For instance, if one answer choice says that quantity x increases and another either says that quantity x decreases (opposite) or says that quantity y increases (parallel), then those answer choices would fall into the same family. An answer choice that doesn't match the construction of the answer choice family is more likely to be incorrect. Most questions will not have answer choice families, but when they do appear, you should be prepared to recognize them.

⊘ Eliminate Answers

Eliminate answer choices as soon as you realize they are wrong, but make sure you consider all possibilities. If you are eliminating answer choices and realize that the last one you are left with is also wrong, don't panic. Start over and consider each choice again. There may be something you missed the first time that you will realize on the second pass.

⊘ Avoid Fact Traps

Don't be distracted by an answer choice that is factually true but doesn't answer the question. You are looking for the choice that answers the question. Stay focused on what the question is asking for so you don't accidentally pick an answer that is true but incorrect. Always go back to the question and make sure the answer choice you've selected actually answers the question and is not merely a true statement.

⊘ Extreme Statements

In general, you should avoid answers that put forth extreme actions as standard practice or proclaim controversial ideas as established fact. An answer choice that states the "process should be used in certain situations, if..." is much more likely to be correct than one that states the "process should be discontinued completely." The first is a calm rational statement and doesn't even make a definitive, uncompromising stance, using a hedge word *if* to provide wiggle room, whereas the second choice is far more extreme.

11

⊘ Benchmark

As you read through the answer choices and you come across one that seems to answer the question well, mentally select that answer choice. This is not your final answer, but it's the one that will help you evaluate the other answer choices. The one that you selected is your benchmark or standard for judging each of the other answer choices. Every other answer choice must be compared to your benchmark. That choice is correct until proven otherwise by another answer choice beating it. If you find a better answer, then that one becomes your new benchmark. Once you've decided that no other choice answers the question as well as your benchmark, you have your final answer.

⊘ Predict the Answer

Before you even start looking at the answer choices, it is often best to try to predict the answer. When you come up with the answer on your own, it is easier to avoid distractions and traps because you will know exactly what to look for. The right answer choice is unlikely to be word-for-word what you came up with, but it should be a close match. Even if you are confident that you have the right answer, you should still take the time to read each option before moving on.

General Strategies

⊘ Tough Questions

If you are stumped on a problem or it appears too hard or too difficult, don't waste time. Move on! Remember though, if you can quickly check for obviously incorrect answer choices, your chances of guessing correctly are greatly improved. Before you completely give up, at least try to knock out a couple of possible answers. Eliminate what you can and then guess at the remaining answer choices before moving on.

⊘ Check Your Work

Since you will probably not know every term listed and the answer to every question, it is important that you get credit for the ones that you do know. Don't miss any questions through careless mistakes. If at all possible, try to take a second to look back over your answer selection and make sure you've selected the correct answer choice and haven't made a costly careless mistake (such as marking an answer choice that you didn't mean to mark). This quick double check should more than pay for itself in caught mistakes for the time it costs.

⊘ Pace Yourself

It's easy to be overwhelmed when you're looking at a page full of questions; your mind is confused and full of random thoughts, and the clock is ticking down faster than you would like. Calm down and maintain the pace that you have set for yourself. Especially as you get down to the last few minutes of the test, don't let the small numbers on the clock make you panic. As long as you are on track by monitoring your pace, you are guaranteed to have time for each question.

⊘ Don't Rush

It is very easy to make errors when you are in a hurry. Maintaining a fast pace in answering questions is pointless if it makes you miss questions that you would have gotten right otherwise. Test writers like to include distracting information and wrong answers that seem right. Taking a little extra time to avoid careless mistakes can make all the difference in your test score. Find a pace that allows you to be confident in the answers that you select.

⊘ KEEP MOVING

Panicking will not help you pass the test, so do your best to stay calm and keep moving. Taking deep breaths and going through the answer elimination steps you practiced can help to break through a stress barrier and keep your pace.

Final Notes

The combination of a solid foundation of content knowledge and the confidence that comes from practicing your plan for applying that knowledge is the key to maximizing your performance on test day. As your foundation of content knowledge is built up and strengthened, you'll find that the strategies included in this chapter become more and more effective in helping you quickly sift through the distractions and traps of the test to isolate the correct answer.

Now that you're preparing to move forward into the test content chapters of this book, be sure to keep your goal in mind. As you read, think about how you will be able to apply this information on the test. If you've already seen sample questions for the test and you have an idea of the question format and style, try to come up with questions of your own that you can answer based on what you're reading. This will give you valuable practice applying your knowledge in the same ways you can expect to on test day.

Good luck and good studying!

Safety and Compliance

Legal and Professional Considerations

ROLE OF LABORATORY PROFESSIONALS IN CUSTOMER SERVICE/SUPPORT

All laboratory professionals serve a role in customer service and support to some degree because they represent the organization with every patient contact, and the patient's attitude toward the organization may be based on this contact. The three components in any delivery of service are the customer (patient, family member, or visitor), the organization (laboratory, hospitals), and the individual service provider (lab professional). For this reason, it is important that the individual remain professional, showing respect and consideration for the patient and others, maintaining a professional appearance, and carrying out duties competently. Communication is the essential element in customer service, including both conveying information in language appropriate to the listener and being an active listener. The laboratory professional should try to anticipate patient concerns, provide reassurance, and answer any questions in a positive, straightforward manner. Body language and words should both convey sincerity, and the laboratory professional should always handle complaints in a positive manner.

INTERPERSONAL COMMUNICATION WITH NON-LABORATORY PERSONNEL

Interpersonal communication skills are essential for the laboratory professional, who must interact with a variety of non-laboratory personnel in the work environment. Elements of effective communication include:

- Showing respect and consideration to others in all communications
- Recognizing each individual's scope of practice and responsibilities toward the patient
- Being an active listener, paying attention, and asking clarifying questions as necessary
- Sharing important information with the appropriate personnel
- Asking questions when in need of more information about a patient
- Ensuring that information is shared accurately
- Providing timely communication
- Discussing special needs of patients in relation to collection of a sample and processing
- Communicating any problems encountered with collection or processing with the appropriate personnel
- Discussing timing issues related to sample collection, such as STAT orders or collection that must be done at a specific time
- Scheduling collection to avoid interrupting other patient care activities when possible

MEDICARE HEALTH PLANS

Medicare Health Plans include managed care plans such as Medicare Advantage, cost plans, or health care prepayment plans. Services provided by contract providers (those who participate in these plans) are reimbursed by Medicare. However, non-contract providers (those outside of these plans who provide services to enrollees (patients), such as a laboratory) may not be reimbursed. If Medicare denies payment to a non-contract provider, that provider must receive notice regarding the reason for the denial and the steps to appeal the decision. The filing for reconsideration must be done within 60 days from the date of notification and must include a signed **waiver of liability** form. The form contains the enrollees Medicare number and name, the name of the non-contract provider, the dates of service, and the name of the health plan. The waiver of liability statement

15

waives any right to collect payment for the services provided regardless of the outcome of the appeal process, although the provider maintains the right to further appeal.

LIABILITY

Liability is legal responsibility for something an individual has done or failed to do. Elements of liability include:

- **Neglect**: Failure to provide basic needs or usual standards of care or exhibiting an uncaring attitude toward a patient
- **Abandonment**: A unilateral severing of the professional relationship between the healthcare provider and the patient with no notice that would allow the patient to make other arrangements
- **Assault**: A threat to touch another person against the patient's will, such as threatening to withdraw blood from an uncooperative patient
- **Battery**: Following through with a threat and touching another person without consent, such as forcing the patient to undergo venipuncture
- **Tort**: Negligent act that causes injury or suffering to another person and is the basis for a civil action, such as a lawsuit
- **Malpractice**: Failure to meet standards of care or wrongfully carrying out duties in such a way as to bring harm to a patient

PATIENT CONSENT

Patients should provide **informed consent** prior to any procedures, including laboratory tests. That is, the patient should understand the purpose, the risks, and the benefits as well as the method that will be used in the procedure. Hospitalized patients sign a general consent form that covers most routine laboratory tests, although some tests, such as HIV tests, may require a separate consent form. While consent may be verbal or in writing, written consent provides the most protection for the healthcare provider. Competent adult patients have the **right to refuse any treatment**, even if it is lifesaving. If a patient refuses a test (for example, a blood draw), the phlebotomist must immediately stop, inform the ordering healthcare provider, and document the refusal.

TYPES OF PATIENT CONSENT

The types of patient consents include the following:

- **Informed consent**: A competent person is able to provide voluntary permission for a medical procedure after receiving adequate information about the risk of, methods used, and consequences of the procedure.
- **Expressed consent**: Permission that is given by patient verbally or in writing for a procedure
- **Implied consent**: The patient's actions imply permission for the procedure without verbal or written consent, for example going to the emergency room to receive care or holding out an arm when told of the need to draw blood.
- **HIV consent**: Special permission must be granted to administer a test for detecting the human immunodeficiency virus.
- **Parental consent for minors**: A parent or a legal guardian must give permission for procedures administered to underage patients. Depending on the state law, patient may be considered underage if they are younger than 21 or younger than 18.

Laboratory Standards and Regulations

OCCUPATIONAL SAFETY AND HEALTH ADMINISTRATION (OSHA)

OSHA stands for Occupational Safety and Health Administration. It is an organization designed to assure the safety and health of workers by setting and enforcing standards; providing training, outreach, and education; establishing partnerships; and encouraging continual improvement in workplace safety and health.

SDS (formerly MSDS) stands for **Safety Data Sheets**. These sheets are the result of the "Right to Know" Law also known as the OSHA's Hazard Communication Standard (HCS). This law requires chemical manufacturers to supply SDS sheets on any products that have a hazardous warning label. These sheets contain information on precautionary as well as emergency information about the product.

OSHA REGULATIONS REGARDING LABORATORY SERVICES

The Occupational Safety and Health Administration (OSHA) requires that facilities provide safe medical equipment and devices. OSHA also regulates workplace safety, including disposal methods for sharps, such as needles, and blood disposition. OSHA requires that standard precautions be used at all times and that staff be trained to use precautions. OSHA requires procedures for post-exposure evaluation and treatment and availability of hepatitis B vaccine for healthcare workers. OSHA defines occupational exposure to infections, establishes standards to prevent the spread of bloodborne pathogens, and regulates the fitting and use of respirators. OSHA requires the use of needleless blood transfer devices as a means of decreasing the risk of needlestick injuries and infection as part of OSHA's Bloodborne Pathogen Standard. Sharps used for blood draw should have sharps injury protection devices whenever possible. Needles without this protection should never be recapped as this increases risk of needlestick. States may have their own OSHA-approved programs but must meet the minimum standards developed by OSHA.

LABORATORY STANDARDS AND INTEGRITY ASSESSMENT

Laboratory standards are established by a number of agencies, including OSHA, which establishes safety standards; the EPA, which established good laboratory practices; CLSI, which provides global laboratory standards; and ISO-9000, which establishes standards for quality management. Laboratory standards are norms or requirements stablished for the profession. **Integrity assessment** is carried out to determine if a laboratory is meeting standards or has engaged in fraud or misconduct (as opposed to accidents or errors), such as through:

- Failure to properly carry out procedures
- Falsification of records or measurements, incomplete documentation, manipulation of data
- Violation of standards or rules of conduct, violations of codes of ethics
- Misrepresentation of quality assurance results
- Failure to adequately calibrate equipment
- Failure to retain samples for the required time
- Improper storage of reagents, samples, and supplies
- Failure to follow standard operating procedures
- Alterations of log book
- Employment of personnel without appropriate license or certification

Integrity assessment may include reviewing data, comparing manual logs with computer logs, conducting an audit trail, carrying out unannounced audits, and encouraging and supporting whistleblowers.

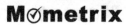

GOVERNMENTAL AND NONGOVERNMENTAL REGULATORY ENTITIES

The **Clinical and Laboratory Standards Institute (CLSI)** provides standards for a wide range of performance and testing and covers all types of laboratory functions and microbiology. These standards are used as a basis for quality control procedures. Standards include: labeling, security/information technology, toxicology/drug testing, statistical quality control, and performance standards for various types of antimicrobial susceptibility testing.

In the United States, all laboratory testing, except for research, is regulated by the CMS (Centers for Medicare and Medicaid) through **Clinical Laboratory Improvement Amendments (CLIA)**. CLIA is implemented through the Division of Laboratory Services and serves approximately 244,000 laboratories. Laboratories receiving reimbursement from CMS must meet CLIA standards, which ensure that laboratory testing will be accurate and procedures followed properly.

The **Centers for Disease Control and Prevention (CDC)** is a federal agency that supports health promotion, prevention, and health preparedness. The CDC partners with CMS and the FDA in supporting CLIA programs.

The **National Accrediting Agency for Clinical Laboratory Sciences** is responsible for approving and accrediting clinical laboratory science and similar healthcare professional education programs.

The **College of American Pathologists** is the primary organization for board-certified pathologists serving to represent the interests of the public, as well as pathologists and their patients by fostering excellence in the pathology and laboratory medicine practice.

The **Joint Commission** is a large organization that aims to improve the quality of care provided to patients through implementing healthcare accreditation standards and other supportive services aimed at improving the performance of healthcare organizations.

SOP FOR LABORATORIES

Each laboratory should draw up a **standard operating procedure (SOP) document** that outlines all the processes and procedures associated with the reception of a sample and processing, including:

- **Specimen collection processes**: PPE, patient identification, collection tubes, collecting procedures, need for special handling, labeling, transporting specimens, criteria for rejecting inadequate sample, protocols for adverse reactions
- **Chain of custody**: Labeling, storing, packing, and transporting
- **Sample reception**: Specimen identification, logging, specimen condition, specimen accountability, retention times
- **Rejection criteria**: Incorrect collection tube, leaking tube, incorrect labeling, incorrect sample for test, volume inadequate, order unverified, mismatch between order and labeling
- **Delivery** (from reception to processing): Process for delivery to correct department, specimen retention policies
- **Processing**: Procedures for testing, accountability standards, storage, and retention policies
- **Reporting**: Methods of reporting and timeframes

Laboratory Safety and Quality Control

QUALITY IMPROVEMENT

Quality improvement is a systematic method of analyzing performance and improving the quality of performance, usually across an entire organization although more localized quality improvement methods may be employed. Methods of quality improvement include:

- **Continuous Quality Improvement** (CQI): Emphasizes the organization and systems and processes within that organization rather than individuals. It recognizes internal customers (staff) and external customers (patients) and utilizes data to improve processes.
- **Total Quality Management** (TQM): Espouses a commitment to meeting the needs of the customers at all levels within an organization, promoting not only continuous improvement but also a dedication to quality in all aspects of an organization. Outcomes should include increased customer satisfaction, productivity, and increased profits through efficiency and reduction in costs.
- **Six Sigma®**: A data-driven performance model that aims to eliminate "defects" in processes that involve products or services. The first model for Six Sigma® is DMAIC (define, measure, analyze, improve, control) and is used when existing processes or products need improvement and is utilized in healthcare quality.

PHILOSOPHY OF CONTINUOUS QUALITY IMPROVEMENT

Continuous quality improvement is a multidisciplinary management philosophy that can be applied to all aspects of an organization, whether related to such varied areas as the cardiac unit, purchasing, laboratories, or human resources. The skills used for epidemiologic research (data collection, analysis, outcomes, action plans) are all applicable to analysis of multiple types of events because they are based on solid scientific methods. Multi-disciplinary planning can bring valuable insights from various perspectives, and strategies used in one context can often be applied to another. All staff, from housekeeping to supervising, must be alert to not only problems but also opportunities for improvement. Increasingly, departments must be concerned with cost-effectiveness as the costs of medical care continue to rise, so the quality professional in the cardiovascular unit is not in an isolated position in an institution but is just one part of the whole, facing similar concerns as those in other disciplines. Disciplines are often interrelated in their functions.

DEMING'S 14 POINTS FOR QUALITY IMPROVEMENT

- Create and communicate to all employees a statement of the quality philosophy of the company.
- Adopt this philosophy.
- Build quality into a product throughout production.
- End the practice of awarding business on the basis of price tag alone and build a long-term relationship based on established loyalty and trust.
- Work to constantly improve quality and productivity.
- Institute on-the-job quality training.
- Teach and institute leadership to improve all job functions.
- Drive out fear, create trust.
- Strive to reduce inter- and intradepartmental conflicts.
- Eliminate slogans and targets. Instead, focus on the system and morale.
- Eliminate numerical quotas for production and management. Substitute leadership methods for improvement.
- Remove barriers that rob people of pride in their work.
- Educate with self-improvement programs.
- Include everyone in the company to accomplish the transformation.

RISK MANAGEMENT

Risk management attempts to prevent harm and legal liability by being proactive and by identifying a patient's **risk factors**. The patient should be educated about these factors and ways that they can modify their behavior to decrease their risk. Treatments and interventions must be considered in terms of risk to the patient, and the patient must always know these risks in order to make healthcare decisions. Much can be done to avoid mistakes that put patients at risk. Patients should note medications, allergies, and other aspects of their care so that they can help prevent mistakes. They should feel free to question care and to have their concerns heard and addressed. When mistakes are made, the actions taken to remedy the situation are very important. The physician or nurse should be made aware of the error immediately, and the patient notified according to hospital policy. Errors must be evaluated to determine how the process failed. Honesty and caring can help mitigate many errors.

Laboratory Infection Control

CHAIN OF INFECTION

In order for an infection to spread it requires an agent, a host, and the proper environment (known as the epidemiologic triad). The **chain of infection** takes that model a step further, stating that in order for a pathogenic microorganism to leave its original reservoir (which could be an animal, a human, or the environment) it needs a portal of exit from that reservoir, a susceptible host to inhabit, a mode of transmission between reservoir and host, and a portal of entry into the host.

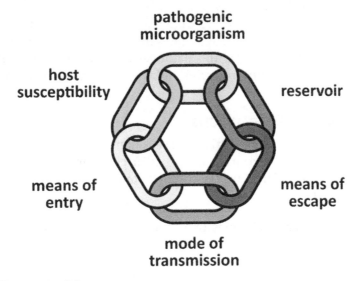

BASIC INFECTION CONTROL MEASURES

Standard infection control measures are designed to prevent transmission of microbial substances between patients and/or medical providers. These measures are indicated for everyone and include frequent handwashing, gloves whenever bodily fluids are involved, and face shields and gowns when splashes are anticipated. For more advanced control with tuberculosis, SARS, vesicular rash disorders (such as VZV), and more recently COVID-19, **airborne precautions** should be instituted to prevent the spread of tiny droplets that can remain suspended in the air for days and travel throughout a hospital environment. Therefore, negative pressure rooms are essential, and providers and patients should wear high-efficiency N95 masks and be fitted in advance. For disorders such as influenza or other infections spread by droplets (spread by cough or sneeze) **droplet precautions** such as wearing basic surgical masks must be taken. For **contact precautions** in the setting of fecally-transmitted infection or vesicular rash diseases, gowns/gloves should be used and contact limited. White coats are not a substitute for proper gowning.

21

DIRECT AND INDIRECT CONTACT TRANSMISSION

According to the CDC, contact transmission is the most common form of disease transmission. Organisms commonly spread through contact include herpes simplex, *Clostridium difficile*, and *Staphylococcus aureus*. Types of contact transmission:

- **Direct contact**: Transmission is directly from one person to another, usually because of touch. Examples include a person's blood or other body fluids entering broken skin, mucous membranes, or cuts of another person (such as with HIV) and mites (such as scabies) from one person transferring to another's skin.
- **Indirect contact**: Transmission occurs from one person, through an intermediary object or person, and then to another person. Examples include when a caregiver's hands touch a patient or bedrails contaminated with a pathogen and then pass that pathogen to a third person (such as with *Clostridium difficile*), and when patient care devices or other items are shared among different patients.

PROPER INFECTION CONTROL PRECAUTIONS

Each laboratory should carry out a biological risk assessment every year or when new risks arise to determine the biosafety level, agent hazards, and procedures hazards. Work practices should conform to Bloodborne Pathogen Standard (OSHA) and standard precautions (CDC). **Infection control precautions** include:

- Utilizing appropriate hand hygiene with a hands-free sink for washing hands available near exit
- Using mechanical pipettes instead of mouth pipetting
- Prohibiting eating, drinking, smoking, storing food, applying makeup, and handling contact lenses in the laboratory
- Maintaining safe handling of sharps policies
- Utilizing safety devices (retractable needles, lances) when possible
- Minimizing splashing or aerosolizing liquids
- Decontaminating potentially infectious materials prior to disposal
- Packing potentially infectious materials for disposal outside of the facility in appropriate packaging according to regulations
- Maintaining a pest management program
- Ensuring all personnel are adequately trained
- Ensuring appropriate immunizations and screening for personnel
- Making PPE available and monitoring appropriate use
- Ensuring eye wash station is easily accessed and available

SPECIFIC INFECTION PREVENTION AND CONTROL
HEPATITIS B

Hepatitis B virus and its exposure hazards are discussed below:

- Hepatitis B is a sexually transmitted infection, also transmitted with body fluids.
- Some individuals may be symptom free but still be carriers.
- Condoms are not proven to prevent the spread of this disease.
- Symptoms include jaundice, dark urine, malaise, joint pain, fever, fatigue.
- Labs will show decreased albumin levels, positive hepatitis B antibodies and antigens, and increased levels of transaminase.
- For treatment, monitor for changes in the liver. Recombinant alpha interferon may be used in some cases. Transplant is necessary if liver failure occurs.
- Prevention involves a series of 3 Hepatitis B Vaccinations: an initial dose, a dose 1 month later, and a final dose 6 months after the initial dose.
- HBV is the most common laboratory-associated infection.

HEPATITIS D

The hepatitis D virus is the most severe form of hepatitis that occurs in the presence of hepatitis B. Its exposure hazards are discussed below:

- Hepatitis D is also referred to as delta hepatitis and involves severe infection of the liver. It requires hepatitis B to replicate and therefore occurs as a super infection with hepatitis B. Without hepatitis B, hepatitis D cannot thrive.
- Signs and symptoms include jaundice, fatigue, abdominal pain, loss of appetite, nausea, vomiting, joint pain, and dark (tea colored) urine.
- Transmission occurs when blood from an infected person enters the body of a person who is not immune. This can happen through sharing drugs, needles, or "works" when "shooting" drugs; through needle sticks or sharps exposures on the job; or from an infected mother to her baby during birth. Activation and replication of hepatitis D then occurs in the individual with hepatitis B.
- Treatment for acute HDV infection involves supportive care. Treatment for chronic HDV infection involves interferon-alfa and liver transplant.
- Because hepatitis D requires hepatitis B to replicate, prevention of hepatitis D is through the prevention of HBV with hepatitis B vaccination. For individuals already with HBV, prevention of hepatitis D is through education to reduce high-risk behaviors and avoid transmission.

HIV

The following are ways that HIV can be **transmitted** from an infected person to an uninfected one:

- HIV can be transmitted through **direct blood contact**, including injection drug needles, blood transfusions, accidents in health care settings, or use of certain blood products.
- **Sexual intercourse (vaginal and anal)**: In the genitals and the rectum, HIV may infect the mucous membranes directly or enter through cuts and sores caused during intercourse (many of which would be unnoticed).
- **Oral sex** (mouth-penis, mouth-vagina): The mouth is an inhospitable environment for HIV (HIV is more often found in semen, vaginal fluid, or blood), meaning the risk of HIV transmission through the throat, gums, and oral membranes is lower than through vaginal or anal membranes. There are, however, documented cases where HIV was transmitted orally.
- **Sharing injection needles**: An injection needle can pass blood directly from one person's bloodstream to another. It is a very efficient way to transmit a blood-borne virus.
- **Mother to child**: It is possible for an HIV-infected mother to pass the virus directly before or during birth, or through breast milk. The following "bodily fluids" are NOT infectious: saliva, tears, sweat, feces, and urine.

PROTOCOL FOR NEEDLESTICK INJURY

If the phlebotomist experiences a needlestick injury after carrying out a venipuncture, the phlebotomist's initial response should be to wash the wound with soap and water. As soon as possible, the incident must be reported to a supervisor and steps taken according to established protocol. This may include testing and/or prophylaxis, depending on the patient's health history. In some cases, the patient may also be tested for communicable diseases, such as HIV, in order to determine the risk to the phlebotomist. PEP (post-exposure prophylaxis) is available for exposure to HIV (human immunodeficiency virus) and HBV (hepatitis B virus). However, no PEP is available for HCV (hepatitis C virus) although the CDC does provide a plan for management. PEP should be initiated within 72 hours of exposure. All testing and treatments associated with the needlestick injury must be provided free of cost to the phlebotomist.

DONNING AND DOFFING PROTECTIVE CLOTHING

A healthcare worker puts on (dons) the protective gown first, being sure not to touch the outside of the gown. The mask is put on next. Gloves are applied last and secured over the cuffs of the gown. When doffing (taking off) protective clothing, a healthcare worker removes the gloves first. They are removed by grasping one glove at the wrist and pulling it inside out, off the hand, and holding it in the gloved hand. The second glove is removed by placing the uncovered hand's fingers under the edge of the glove, being careful not to touch the outside of the glove, and rolling it down inside out over the glove grasped in the gloved hand. The first glove ends up inside of the second glove. Next slide arms out of the gown and then fold the gown with the outside folded away from the body so that the contaminated side is folded inwardly. Dispose of properly. Finally, remove the mask by touching the strings only. Always wash hands after glove removal

Laboratory Hazards

BIOLOGICAL/BIOHAZARDOUS AND HAZARDOUS WASTE

Biological wastes are those that contain or are contaminated with pathogens (human, plant, animal); rDNA; blood, cell, or tissue products; and cultures. Biological wastes that are, or may, be infectious or rDNA contaminated (biohazardous waste) must be inactivated before disposal in hazardous waste containers. Typically, inactivation is carried out with autoclaving or treating with hypochlorite solution (bleach). Contaminated sharps must be maintained in special sharps containers to avoid injury to handlers, and inactivated before disposal. Non-infectious biological wastes, such as uncontaminated gloves, do not require deactivation and are disposed of in biological waste containers. **Hazardous wastes**, those that are ignitable, corrosive, reactive, or toxic, are any that are harmful to humans or the environment and may be solids, liquids, solid gases, or sludges. Hazardous wastes are generally transported by hazardous waste transporters in special hazardous waste containers to Treatment Storage and Disposal Facilities (TSDFs) where they are stored, inactivated, and/or recycled.

Biohazard Symbol

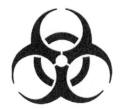

ROUTES BIOLOGICAL HAZARDS MAY TAKE TO ENTER THE BODY

Biological hazards may enter the body through the following avenues:

- Airborne (through the nasal passage into the lungs)
- Ingestion (by eating)
- Broken Skin
- Percutaneous (through intact skin)
- Mucosal (through the lining of the mouth and nose)

CLEANING UP SMALL BLOOD SPILLS

The best way to clean a small blood spill is to absorb the blood with a paper towel or gauze pad. Then disinfect the area with a disinfectant. Soap and water are not considered a disinfectant nor is alcohol. Never scrape a dry spill; this may cause an aerosol of infectious organisms. If blood is dried, use the disinfectant to moisten the dried blood.

BIOTERRORISM

Bioterrorism is the use of biological agents (viruses, bacteria, fungi) to attack and cause illness, death, or contamination in people, air supplies, water supplies, animals, and/or crops. There are similar steps to take regardless of the pathogen. An organized approach should include the following steps:

- Be on the alert for possible bioterrorism-related infections, based on clusters of patients or symptoms.
- Use personal protection equipment, including respirators when indicated.
- Complete a thorough assessment of the patient, including medical history, physical examination, immunization record, and travel history.
- The physician should give a probable diagnosis based on symptoms and lab findings, including cultures.
- Healthcare staff should provide treatment, including prophylaxis while waiting for laboratory findings.
- Use transmission precautions as well as isolation for suspected biologic agents.
- Notify local, state, and federal authorities as per established protocol.
- Conduct surveillance and epidemiological studies to identify at risk populations.
- Healthcare facilities should develop plans to accommodate large numbers of patients, such as:
  - Restricting elective admissions
  - Transferring patients to other facilities
  - Reutilizing existing facilities

PROTOCOL FOR THE DISPOSAL OF REAGENTS

Laboratories use many different reagent solutions, which comprise a solid (solute) dissolved in a liquid (solvent). The three most common **types of reagents** include:

- **Stock**: Concentrate that is diluted to prepare a working solution
- **Working**: Diluted solution ready for use
- **Standard**: Reference solution used to identify the concentration of other solutions

Reagents may be classified as solid wastes (which can include liquids) or hazardous wastes. Some reagents, such as those containing sodium azide, must be disposed of as hazardous waste in hazardous waste drums and sent to hazardous waste facilities for incineration (most hazardous wastes cannot go into landfills), but some others, such as ethanol diluted to less than 24%, may be discharged into the sewer. Some, such as DAB, may be detoxified before sewer disposal. Manufacturer's directions for disposal must be followed for each reagent.

FIRE SAFETY

Fire requires three components, known as the fire triangle, in order to occur. The fire triangle includes fuel, oxygen, and heat. When a chemical source is included, it is known as the fire tetrahedron. In the event of a fire remember these two acronyms, RACE and PASS. **RACE** describes the steps for dealing with a fire. "R" stands for Rescue (rescue patients and co-workers from danger.) "A" stands for alarm (sound the alarm and alert those around you.) "C" stands for confine (confine a fire by closing the doors and windows.) "E" stands for extinguish (use the nearest fire extinguisher to put out the fire). **PASS** describes how to use a fire extinguisher to put out a fire. "P" stands for pull the pin. "A" stands for aim at the fire. "S" stands for squeeze the trigger. "S" stands for sweep the base of the fire. Fires are broken down into **four classes**:

- Class A fires involve ordinary combustible materials.
- Class B fires involve flammable liquids.
- Class C fires are electrical fires.
- Class D fires involve combustible metals.

Ethics

ETHICAL PRINCIPLES

Autonomy is the ethical principle that the individual has the right to make decisions about his or her own care. In the case of children or patients with dementia who cannot make autonomous decisions, parents or family members may serve as the legal decision maker. The healthcare worker must keep the patient and/or family fully informed so that they can exercise their autonomy in informed decision-making.

Justice is the ethical principle that relates to the distribution of the limited resources of healthcare benefits to the members of society. These resources must be distributed fairly. For example, imagine there is only one bed left and two sick patients. Justice comes into play in deciding which patient should stay and which should be transported or otherwise cared for. The decision should be made according to what is best or most just for the patients and not colored by personal bias.

Beneficence is an ethical principle that involves performing actions that are for the purpose of benefitting another person. In the care of a patient, any procedure or treatment should be done with the ultimate goal of benefitting the patient, and any actions that are not beneficial should be reconsidered. As conditions change, procedures need to be continually reevaluated to determine if they are still of benefit.

Nonmaleficence is an ethical principle that means healthcare workers should provide care in a manner that does not cause direct intentional harm to the patient:

- The actual act must be good or morally neutral.
- The intent must be only for a good effect.
- A bad effect cannot serve as the means to get to a good effect.
- A good effect must have more benefit than a bad effect has harm.

SCOPE OF PRACTICE AND ETHICAL STANDARDS RELATED TO PRACTICE OF PHLEBOTOMY

The **scope of practice** encompasses those duties and procedures that the person's training, licensure and/or certification has prepared the person to undertake. The phlebotomist and other laboratory professionals must adhere to the **code of ethics** developed by the American Society for Clinical Laboratory Sciences (ASCLS):

- **Duty to patient**: This is the primary focus and depends on being honest, showing respect for the patient, and providing a high standard of care.
- **Duty to colleagues and profession**: The phlebotomist and laboratory professionals must establish an honest and cooperative working relationship with colleagues and work to improve personal practice and to advance the profession.
- **Duty to society**: The phlebotomist and laboratory professionals must comply with laws and regulations and serve as patient advocates.
- **Pledge**: The phlebotomist and laboratory professionals pledge to carry out the duties outlined in the code of ethics, beginning with placing the welfare of the patient before that of self.

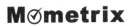

BIOETHICS

Bioethics is a branch of ethics that involves making sure that the medical treatment given is the most morally correct choice given the different options that might be available and the differences inherent in the varied levels of treatment. In the health care unit, if the patients, family members, and the staff are in agreement when it comes to values and decision-making, then no ethical dilemma exists; however, when there is a difference in value beliefs between the patients/family members and the staff, there is a bioethical dilemma that must be resolved. Sometimes, discussion and explanation can resolve differences, but at times the institution's ethics committee must be brought in to resolve the conflict. The primary goal of bioethics is to determine the most morally correct action using the set of circumstances given.

ETHICAL ANALYSIS OF A SITUATION

Assessment of the situation is done to reveal the **ethical, legal, and professional conflicts** that are present. Those who are involved are identified, including the patient, family, and healthcare personnel. The decision-maker is determined if it is not the patient. Information about the situation is collected to determine medical facts about the disease and condition of the patient, options for treatment, and diagnoses. Any pertinent legal information is included. The patient and family's cultural, religious, and moral values are determined. Possible courses of action are listed and compared in terms of outcomes for the patient using the utilitarian or deontological theory of ethics. Professional codes of ethics are also applied. A decision is made and evaluated as to whether it is the most morally correct action. Ethical arguments for and against the decision are given and responded to by the decision-maker.

PATIENT RIGHTS AND RESPONSIBILITIES

Empowering patients and families to act as their own advocates requires they have a clear understanding of their **rights and responsibilities**. These should be given (in print form) and/or presented (audio/video) to patients and families on admission or as soon as possible:

- **Rights** should include competent, non-discriminatory medical care that respects privacy and allows participation in decisions about care and the right to refuse care. They should have clear, understandable explanations of treatments, options, and conditions, including outcomes. They should be apprised of transfers, changes in care plan, and advance directives. They should have access to medical records information about charges.
- **Responsibilities** should include providing honest and thorough information about health issues and medical history. They should ask for clarification if they don't understand information that is provided to them, and they should follow the plan of care that is outlined or explain why that is not possible. They should treat staff and other patients with respect.

> **Review Video: <u>Patient Advocacy</u>**
> Visit mometrix.com/academy and enter code: 202160

Patient Preparation

Introduction and Patient Identification

INITIATING PATIENT CONTACT

When initiating patient contact prior to conducting specimen collection, the following procedures should be followed:

1. Knock on the door before entering the patient's room, slowly open the door, and ask if it is alright to enter.
2. Look for signs on the door indicating special precautions that must be taken (e.g., protective clothing needed).
3. Identify your name and reason for entering room.
4. In the event of a physician or member of the clergy being in the room, it may still be appropriate to explain who you are and proceed to do the draw if the draw is STAT.
5. If the patient is verbal, inquire about any issues (e.g., a history of fainting during venipuncture) or preferences (e.g., having family remain in the room vs. asking them to leave, telling the patient when the needle is about to be inserted vs. not telling them) they might have for the procedure.

IDENTIFYING THE PATIENT

The first step in any blood draw or laboratory procedure for inpatients and outpatients should be to properly **identify the patient**, utilizing at least two forms of identification. Alert and responsive patients (or parents of a minor) may be asked to give their names and birthdates:

- Introduce oneself to the patient and explain one's purpose.
- Check ID band against information provided by the patient/caregiver/parent.
- Match specimen labeling to information on the ID band and label immediately with barcode labeler or permanent ink.
- Check ankles for an ID band if it is missing from wrists.
- Consider only the ID bands actually on the patient as valid (not on bedside stand/bed) except in special circumstances (severe burns of extremities). Verify ID with nurse in these cases.
- If armband is missing, procure an armband and secure it on patient before the procedure.
- Ask outpatients for a picture ID and verify the name and birthdate verbally if possible.
- For emergent situations (unconscious patient in ED), check "Jane/John Doe" ID as per protocol.
- For call reports, verify the patient's name, birthdate, and ID number.

COMMUNICATING WITH A PATIENT

Prior to collecting a sample, it is important to make introductions to the patient, check the patient's identification, often through asking name and birthdate and checking wristband, and explain the purpose of the visit ("My name is John Doe, and I'm going to draw blood for the thyroid tests that your physician has ordered"). The phlebotomist should make a point of explaining actions ("I'm going to take a look at the veins in your arms") and should ask if the patient has a preference, ("Where do you prefer to have blood drawn?") if possible. If patients, especially young children, are quite nervous or frightened, chatting with them briefly may help to distract them. The phlebotomist should remain professional and confident throughout the procedure and avoid making statements that may not be true (e.g., "You will barely feel this") because this violates the trust between the patient and phlebotomist.

PATIENT INTERVIEW

Interviewing strategies and techniques include:

- Establishing rapport with the patient: Take time to make introductions and talk for a moment, especially if the patient appears anxious.
- Positioning within the patient's field of vision: Position yourself face-to-face with the patient so that the patient does not have to look up or down during the interview.
- Avoiding medical jargon: Ask questions and respond in language that the patient is familiar with and explain any unclear terms used.
- Ensuring patient privacy/confidentiality: Be alert to the surroundings and make sure that questions and patient's responses remain confidential and cannot be overheard.
- Observing body language: Note nonverbal communication (eye contact, gestures, position, expressions, proxemics) for clues about the patient's emotional state and feelings.
- Asking open-ended questions: Avoid questions that can be answered with a simple "yes" or "no" as much as possible.
- Allowing patient time to respond: Do not look at a watch, fidget, or appear in a hurry.
- Practicing active listening: Make eye contact, nod, respond, and pay attention when patient speaks.
- Respecting cultural differences: Avoid judgmental attitudes or comments.

Laboratory Orders

WRITTEN ORDERS FOR TESTS

Written and signed orders must be received for all tests, so telephone orders or verbal orders (such as in emergency situations) must be followed by a signed written order, which can be delivered, mailed, or electronically submitted to the laboratory. Tests may be ordered by the physician, the advanced practice nurse (such as a nurse practitioner,) or the physician's assistant caring for the patient. The ordering healthcare provider must document in the patient's record the intention of having the test performed and the medical necessity for the test. Written orders should contain the date ordered, the time the test should be carried out, and the diagnostic code (ICD-10-CM) for each test ordered. The order should be appropriate for the diagnostic code, or CMS and insurance companies may not reimburse for the cost of the test.

ADD-ON REQUESTS

Add-on requests are tests ordered on the same sample after the original laboratory test is completed. Add-on requests, as all laboratory orders, must be received in writing, paper or electronic. The add-on requests may be part of the original order indicating that if a test result is abnormal, then one or more additional tests should be carried out. The add-on test may also be ordered once the original test results are received. Add-on requests should indicate the sample that the add-on applies to. Some considerations include:

- Length of time the specimens are saved
- Storage: Refrigerated, room temperature, or frozen
- Specimen viability
- Adequacy of sample

For example, if a hematology sample is kept at room temperature, some tests, such as CBC, can be carried out within 24 hours of collection time. Some tests (such as the reticulocyte count) can be carried out within 24 hours if the sample is refrigerated. Other tests must be conducted within 1-12 hours of collection time, depending on the type of specimen. Some add-on tests should be avoided because the results may be inaccurate, including glucose, potassium, and bilirubin.

REQUISITION FORM

The requisition form is the form in which the tests a patient is having are entered, and the requisition then becomes part of the patient's permanent record. Requisition forms may be filled out manually or electronically. Electronic requisitions often automatically print out the labels with barcodes that will be affixed to the collection tubes. Required elements for a requisition form include the following:

- Name of ordering healthcare provider
- Patient's full name
- Patient's ID number (patient number if an inpatient)
- Room number if inpatient
- Patient's birthdate
- Test to be performed
- Test priorities
- Date and specific directions for test (e.g., "stat" or "fasting")
- Billing information and codes as needed
- Allergies or any special precautions (e.g., "latex allergy" or "sensitive to adhesive")

The laboratory professional should carefully check the requisition to make sure it is complete, verify the patient's identification before proceeding with sample collections, ensure any test requirements, such as "fasting," have been met, verify the date, and determine the priorities for collection.

PATIENT REGISTRATION AND TEST ORDER VERIFICATION

Patient registration requires obtaining information about the patient and entering that information into the records, which are usually in an internal database. The information required includes:

- The patient's name, address, social security number, birth date, telephone number, email address (optional) and the name and telephone number of an emergency contact
- Information about the responsible party. For example, if the patient is a child, the responsible party is generally a parent.
- Information about the policyholder's insurance, both primary and secondary. For example, patients on Medicare provide information about their Medicare coverage as well as any supplementary insurance.

Test order verification requires checking the laboratory order to ensure that it is correctly written, signed, and includes the ICD-10-CM diagnostic code for each order and that each order is appropriate for the diagnosis. For Medicare/Medicaid, verification includes determining whether the test is covered and within the appropriate time frame if it is a repeat test. Some tests may require preauthorization from insurance companies. The laboratory directory may be accessed to determine requirements for testing, such as minimum volume.

SAMPLE REGISTRATION

Sample registration begins with patient registration, which enters identifying information about the patient into the system. If an electronic laboratory information system (LIS) is in use, then labels and barcodes for specimen tubes are generated during patient registration. When the specimen is brought to the laboratory for processing, the sample is registered as part of the existing patient registration by retrieving the patient's file, based on ID number assigned during registration and inputting information. If an LIS is not in use and laboratory records are done manually, labels and barcodes may be generated on arrival at the lab. The sample is assigned a number and the time of the collection, arrival time, and the type of tube and additive are all noted. The location of the sample is tracked, with the record indicating exactly where the sample is placed, such as the shelf, container, row, and number in a refrigerator if the sample is stored.

MINIMUM REQUIREMENTS FOR LABELING SPECIMENS

Laboratory specimens should always be labeled after collection with a label that is permanently attached (with adhesive). The tube or other container should never be labeled in advance, and permanent ink (generally black) should be used for any lettering:

- **Hand-written label**: A label must be hand-written with required information, which must include the patient's full name, ID number (temporary or permanent) if available, date of birth, date and time of specimen collection, and the phlebotomist's signature or initials.
- **Pre-printed label**: If a label is preprinted with the patient's name and other identifying information and/or a barcode, the phlebotomist must attach the label and write the date and time on the letter and sign with signature or initials.

Any special considerations, such as "fasting" should be noted on the label as well. Before the phlebotomist leaves the patient's side, the phlebotomist should compare the label on the specimen to the patient's ID bracelet or record and the laboratory requisition to ensure they all match. Once labeled, the specimen should be placed in a biohazard bag or container for transport.

LABORATORY RESULTS

Information that must be included on the laboratory results includes the name, address, and contact information for the lab, the patient's name, birthdate, gender, and ID number (if one is assigned) and the name of the requesting provider. The results must include the date and time the specimen was collected and the date and time each test result was verified. The tests should be listed along with the value, units, and reference ranges, with some indication of abnormal values, such as high (H) or low (L), abnormal (A), critical high (CH) or critical low (CL). The lab results should be separated by type, such as chemistry panels and hematology panels. Laboratory results may be **distributed to ordering providers** in a number of different ways:

- **Paper**: Results may be delivered by courier, placed in the physician's hospital mailbox, or mailed.
- **Telephone**: Results may be transmitted by phone even when a paper or other type of report is given to ensure that the ordering provider receives the information in a timely manner, especially when there are abnormal results.
- **Messaging/email/electronic**: Results must be delivered over secure lines so that confidentiality is not compromised. Reports may be sent automatically. If patients can access through a patient portal, the ordering provider may need to access the report first and indicate it can be released to the patient, depending on how the system is set up.

Cardiovascular System

CARDIOVASCULAR SYSTEM

LAYERS OF THE HEART

Three layers of tissue form the heart wall. The outer layer of the heart wall is the epicardium, the middle layer is the myocardium, and the inner layer is the endocardium:

- **Epicardium**: The membrane that covers the outside of the heart.
- **Myocardium**: The muscular wall of the heart (the thickest of the three layers of the heart wall) that lies between the inner layer (endocardium) and the outer layer (epicardium).
- **Endocardium**: The membrane lining the inside surface of the heart.

HEART CHAMBERS AND VALVES

There are four chambers of the heart that have valves separating them and regulating a one-way flow of blood between the chambers.

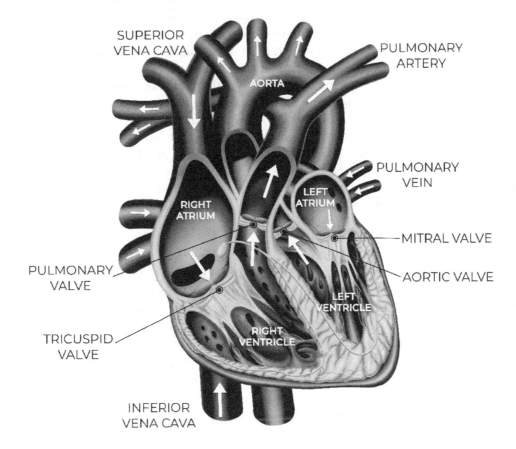

CARDIAC CYCLE

The cardiac cycle consists of ventricular systole and ventricular diastole.

- During **ventricular diastole**, the ventricles relax and the atria contract. Atrial contraction is regulated by the SA node, known as the pacemaker of the heart. The semilunar valves close (causing the "dub" sound) and the atrioventricular valves open, allowing the ventricles to fill.
- During **ventricular systole**, the ventricles contract, which is regulated by the AV node. The semilunar valves (the pulmonic valve and the aortic valve) open, allowing the ventricular contraction to pump blood to the lungs and to the periphery. The atrioventricular valve closes (causing the "lub" sound) to prevent backflow of blood from the ventricles into the atria.

ORIGIN OF HEART SOUNDS

A single heartbeat lasts about one second and consists of a two-part pumping action. As blood collects in both atria (the upper chambers of the heart), the SA node (the heart's natural pacemaker) sends an electrical signal that causes atrial contraction. This contraction forces blood through the mitral and tricuspid valves into the resting ventricles (the lower chambers). This is the longer part of the two-part pumping phase, and it is termed diastole. The pumping phase's second part begins after the ventricles have filled with blood. The electrical impulses from the SA node reach the AV node and then travel to the ventricles, signaling them to contract. This phase is called systole. During ventricular contraction, the mitral and tricuspid valves close tightly to prevent the back flow of blood, but the aortic and pulmonary valves are forced open. Blood ejected from the right ventricle travels to the lungs to get oxygenated. Oxygen-rich blood leaves the left ventricle to travel to all other areas of the body. The ventricles relax, and the pulmonary and aortic valves close after blood enters the aorta and pulmonary artery. The lower pressure in the ventricles causes the tricuspid and mitral valves to open, and the cycle begins again. This system of contractions is repeated, increasing during times of exertion and decreasing while at rest.

ELECTRICAL CONDUCTION SYSTEM

The heart beats (contracts) as a result of **electrical impulses** from the heart muscle (the myocardium). The electrical impulse starts in the **sinoatrial node (SA node)**, which is located in the top of the right atrium. Sometimes the SA node is referred to as the heart's "natural pacemaker." When the SA node releases the electrical signal, the atria contracts. The signal is then passed through the **atrioventricular (AV) node**. After checking the signal, the AV node sends it through ventricular muscle fibers, causing them to contract. The SA node sends electrical impulses at a certain rate, but the heart rate may still change depending on physical demands, stress, or hormonal factors.

ECG Tracing of Cardiac Cycle

ECG tracing of a cardiac cycle is as follows:

- **P wave** represents the atrial depolarization.
- **QRS complex** represents the ventricular depolarization.
- **T wave** represents the ventricular repolarization.

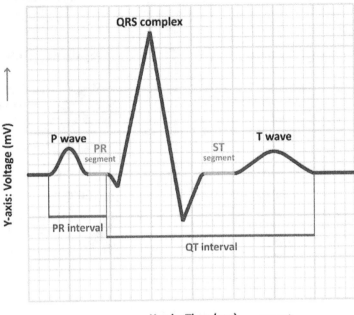

Blood Vessels

The types of blood vessels are described below:

- **Arteries**: Blood vessels that carry blood away from the heart to the body (Arteries do not have valves.)
- **Veins**: Blood vessels that carry the blood from the body back to the heart (Veins have valves.)
- **Capillaries**: One-cell thick blood vessels between arteries and veins that distribute oxygen-rich blood to the body
- **Venules**: The smallest veins
- **Arterioles**: The smallest arteries

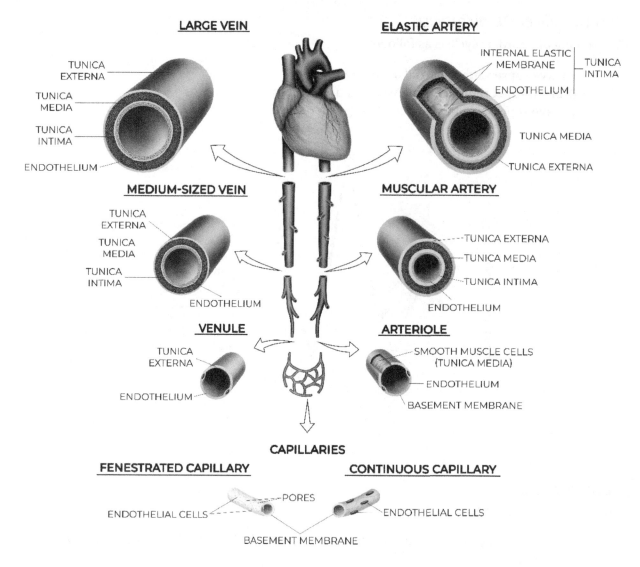

WALLS OF ARTERIES

Wall of an artery consists of three distinct layers of tunics:

- **Tunica intima**: Composed of simple, squamous epithelium called endothelium. Rests on a connective tissue membrane that is rich in elastic and collagenous fibers.
- **Tunica media**: Makes up the bulk of the arterial wall. Includes smooth muscle fibers, which encircle the tube, and a thick layer of elastic connective tissue.
- **Tunica adventitia**: Consists chiefly of connective tissue with irregularly arranged elastic and collagenous fibers. This layer attaches the artery to the surrounding tissues. Also contains minute vessels (vasa vasorum—vessels of vessels) that give rise to capillaries and provide blood to the more external cells of the artery wall.

Smooth muscles in the walls of arteries and arterioles are innervated by the sympathetic branches of the autonomic nervous system. The tunica media and the tunica adventitia are much thicker in arteries.

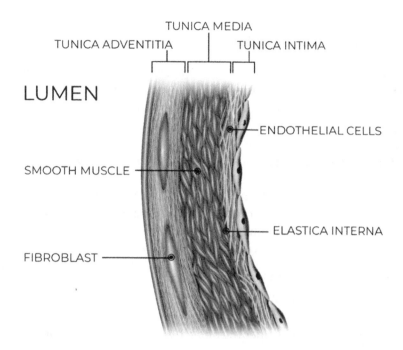

WALLS OF VEINS AND CAPILLARIES

Veins have the same three layers as arteries, but the middle layer is much thinner, so the walls are less muscular and less elastic, and the inner diameter is greater. Some veins, especially those in the arms and legs, contain valves (flaplike) to help prevent backflow. Veins also can serve as blood reservoirs during times of blood loss, constricting to move more blood to the heart.

Capillaries, extensions of the endothelium, are composed of a thin permeable layer of squamous epithelium through which substances in the blood are exchanged for those in tissue.

VEINS OF THE LOWER EXTREMITY

The great saphenous, popliteal, femoral, and lesser saphenous veins are the major **veins** returning blood to the heart from the lower extremities:

- **Great saphenous**: Runs the entire length of the lower extremity and is the longest vein in the body.
- **Popliteal**: Runs deep behind the knee.
- **Femoral**: Runs deep in the upper part of the leg.
- **Lesser saphenous**: Runs lateral to the ankle, up the leg and deep behind the knee.

ARTERIES OF THE UPPER EXTREMITIES

The arteries of the upper extremities are described below:

- **Internal thoracic**: Descends posteriorly to the clavicle's sternal end and enters the thorax
- **Thyrocervical trunk**: Ascends and gives off four different branches, including the transverse and ascending cervical, and suprascapular
- **Suprascapular**: Travels inferolaterally, follows the clavicle in a parallel manner, then goes posteriorly to the scapula
- **Subscapular**: Descends along subscapularis muscle's lateral border to the inferior angle of the scapula
- **Thoracodorsal**: Accompanies the nerve of the same name to the latissimus dorsi muscle
- **Deep brachial**: Accompanies the radial nerve as they pass through the humeral radial groove, then it anastomoses around the elbow joint
- **Ulnar collateral**: Anastomoses around the elbow joint

BLOOD MOVEMENT IN THE CIRCULATORY SYSTEM

The blood flowing through the arterial system is pushed by the pressure built up by the contractions of the heart. The blood flowing through the veins relies on skeletal muscle movement to keep the valves located in the veins opening and closing to keep blood moving toward the heart and not backward through the system.

> **Review Video: Circulatory System**
> Visit mometrix.com/academy and enter code: 376581
>
> **Review Video: Heart Blood Flow**
> Visit mometrix.com/academy and enter code: 783139

VASCULAR SYSTEM FUNCTIONS

The main functions of the vascular system include:

- **Transports** cellular and chemical materials
  - Gases—Oxygen is shuttled to the cells from the lungs and carbon dioxide (a waste product) is transported to the lungs from the cells.
  - Nutrients—In addition to oxygen, other nutrients, like glucose, are transported via the circulatory system. Glucose is shuttled to the liver immediately after digestion. Glucose is used to make ATP (cellular energy), and the liver functions to maintain a stable blood glucose level.
  - Cellular waste—Waste products from digestion, such as ammonia (produced from protein digestion), are transported to the liver to be converted to a less toxic substance, urea, which then moves on to the kidneys and is eventually excreted in the urine.
  - Hormones—The vascular system transports numerous hormones that function to maintain constant internal conditions.
- Contains infection-fighting cells
- Helps stabilize body fluid pH and ionic concentration
- Transports **heat** to help maintain body temperature

BLOOD AND BLOOD COMPONENTS

Blood has numerous functions—gas transport, hemostasis, defense against disease—all of which are brought about by its various components:

- **Red blood cells**: Oxygen transport and gas exchange
- **Blood platelets and coagulation factors**: Coagulation and hemostasis
- **Vitamin K**: Essential cofactor in normal hepatic synthesis of some clotting factors
- **Plasmin**: Lyses fibrin and fibrinogen
- **Antithrombin III**: Inhibits IXa, Xa, XIa, XIIa
- **Complement**: Defense against pyogenic bacteria, activation of phagocytes, clearing of immune complexes, lytic attack on cell membranes
- **Lymphocytes**: Adaptive immune response—killing of specific microbes
- **Monocytes**: Respond to necrotic cell material by migrating to tissues and differentiating into macrophages
- **Neutrophils**: Phagocytosis of microbes
- **Eosinophils**: Phagocytosis, defense against helminthic parasites, allergic reactions
- **Basophils**: Allergic reactions

WHOLE BLOOD, PLASMA, AND SERUM

Whole blood is blood as it is withdrawn from the body. It contains plasma, which includes clotting factors; erythrocytes (red blood cells); leukocytes (white blood cells), which include monocytes, lymphocytes, neutrophils, basophils, and eosinophils; and thrombocytes (platelets). Whole blood is rarely used for testing or administration but is separated into components.

Plasma is the liquid portion of the blood that is free of cells because the erythrocytes, leukocytes, and thrombocytes have been removed. It still contains clotting factors, such as fibrinogen, because it has been treated with an anticoagulant, such as sodium citrate.

Serum, on the other hand, is the liquid portion of blood that is also cell-free but has been allowed to clot and is then spun to separate and remove the clot so that it is also free of clotting factors. Serum is more often used for testing than plasma because serum contains more antigens and can be used for a wider variety of tests. Additionally, anticoagulants found in plasma may interfere with some tests.

RED BLOOD CELLS, WHITE BLOOD CELLS, AND PLATELETS

Blood cells are produced in the bone marrow. Blood is a viscous dark red fluid comprised of cells, gases, and plasma (55%). Blood components include:

- **Erythrocytes** (red blood cells): Red blood cells carry hemoglobin, which transports oxygen. If red blood cell count is low (such as from blood loss) or oxygen carrying capacity is impaired (such as with anemia), the patient may experience hypoxemia (low oxygen). The life cycle is normally 120 days.
- **Leukocytes** (white blood cells): WBCs defend the body against invading organisms (viruses, bacteria, fungi, and parasites) and in the bloodstream and tissues respond to allergies. WBCs include lymphocytes (B, T, natural killer cells, and null cells), monocytes, eosinophils, basophils, and neutrophils.
- **Thrombocytes** (platelets): Platelets release clotting factors and have an active role in forming blood clots.
- **Plasma** (55% of blood): Plasma carries water, proteins, electrolytes, lipids (fats), blood cells, and glucose as well as clotting factors.

41

The primary **blood types** are A, B, AB, and O. Blood is either Rh- or RH+, and patients must receive transfusions of blood that are type and Rh compatible.

OXYGENATION AND OXIDATION OF HEMOGLOBIN

Oxygenation is the loose, reversible binding of hemoglobin (Hgb) with O_2 molecules forming oxyhemoglobin. Hgb oxygenation is the principal method of O_2 uptake from the lungs into the RBCs for transport to the tissues. Each Hgb molecule has the capacity to bind four O_2 molecules since there are four heme molecules in each Hgb. The O_2 binds loosely with the co-ordination bonds of the iron atom in the heme and not the two positive bonds of the iron. Iron is not oxidized and oxygen can be carried to the tissues in the molecular form rather than the ionic form.

Oxidation of Hgb involves the conversion of the functional ferrous (Fe^{2+}) heme iron to the non-functional ferric (Fe^{3+}) form. This is called methemoglobin. This oxidized form of Hgb can't bind or transport oxygen. Oxidation of Hgb may occur due to exposure to toxic chemicals such as nitrites, aniline dyes, and oxidative drugs.

IMMUNOGLOBULIN

Immunoglobulins are proteins created by plasma that attach to foreign substances (bacteria, viruses, etc.), which neutralizes them, and ultimately destroys them. The **types of immunoglobulins** and their functions are explained below:

- **IgA**: Can be located in secretions and prevents viral and bacterial attachment to membranes
- **IgD**: Can be located on B cells and signals for their activation against foreign substances
- **IgE**: The main mediator of mast cells with an allergen exposure
- **IgG**: Primarily found in secondary responses, can cross the placenta, and destroys viruses/bacteria
- **IgM**: Primarily found in first response, located on B cells

ANEMIA

Anemia refers to any condition where there is reduced oxygen carrying capacity due to a fall in hemoglobin concentration with resultant tissue hypoxia. It is defined as Hb <13.5 g/dL in males, <11.5 g/dL in females, <15 g/dL in newborns to three-month-old infants, and <11 g/dL from three months to puberty. Anemia results when compensatory mechanisms fail to restore oxygen levels to meet tissue demands. The following compensatory mechanisms can be seen: arteriolar dilatation, increased cardiac output, increased anaerobic metabolism, increased Hb dissociation, increased erythropoietin output, and internal redistribution of blood flow. If these compensatory mechanisms are adequate, oxygen levels are restored. If not, anemia ensues, with cardiac effects, poor exercise tolerance, lethargy, pallor, headaches, angina on effort, and claudication.

Medical Terminology

ORIGIN OF MEDICAL TERMINOLOGY

Most medical terms derive from Greek or Latin, but there are a few English, French, and German terms. If a Greek or Latin word is broken down into its root, prefix, and suffix, one can understand unfamiliar terminology. To avoid awkward pronunciation when there is no vowel between the root word and suffix, add an -o- to the combining form. For instance, add the suffix *metry* (meaning the measure of) to the root word for eye (*opt*) along with the combining -o- to make the word *optometry*. Examples of English terminology include: Epstein-Barr virus, HIV-positive, 100-mL sample, oxygen-dependent, or self-image. As seen in these examples, English words use a dash instead of a joining vowel. An example of French terminology is *grand mal* (big sickness) for epileptic seizures. An example of German terminology is *mittelschmerz* (middle pain) for the discomfort of ovulation. French and German do not have convenient combining forms, so they must be memorized.

PREFIX, SUFFIX, AND ROOT

Medical terms have three parts:

- **Prefix**: Before the root that modifies the meaning
- **Suffix**: After the root that modifies the meaning
- **Root**: Contains the basic meaning

Examples:

- *Menorrhagia* is excessive bleeding during menstruation and at irregular intervals. The prefix is *meno*, meaning menstruation. The root is *metro*, meaning uterus. The suffix is *rrhagia*, meaning a flow that bursts forth.
- *Rhinoplasty* is a nose job. The root is *rhino*, meaning nose. The suffix is *plasty*, meaning reconstructive surgery.
- *Antecubitum* is the bend of the arm where the nurse draws blood. The root is *cubitum*, meaning elbow. The prefix is *ante*, meaning forward or before.

PREFIXES

Prefix	Meaning	Example
Ab	from, not here, off the norm	Abnormal
Ad	to, in the direction of	Adduct
Ante	prior to, in front of, previously	Antecedent
Anti	hostile to, against, contradictory	Antisocial
Be	make, aligned with, greatly	Benign
Bi	two, occurring twice	Bicycle
De	away, versus, reduce	Deduct
Dia	transverse, across	Diameter
Dis	contradictory, disparate, away	Disjointed
En	create, put in or on, surround	Engulf
Syn	by means of, together, same	Synthesis
Trans	across, far away, go through	Transvaginal
Ultra	extreme, beyond in space	Ultrasound
Un	opposing, antithetical, not	Uncooperative

The following is a list of additional **medical terminology prefixes**:

Prefix	Meaning	Prefix	Meaning
A	without	Multi	numerous
An	without	Neo	new
Bin	two	Nulli	none
Brady	slow	Pan	total
Dys	difficult	Para	beyond
Endo	within	Per	through
Epi	over	Peri	surrounding
Eu	normal	Poly	many
Ex	outward	Post	after
Exo	outward	Pre	before
Hemi	half	Pro	before
Hyper	excessive	Sub	below
Hypo	deficient	Supra	superior
Inter	between	Sym	join
Intra	within	Tachy	rapid
Meta	change	Tetra	four
Micro	minute, tiny	Uni	one

SUFFIXES

Suffix	Meaning	Example
-fication/-ation	manner or process	classification
-gram	written down or illustrated	cardiogram
-graph	a machine or instrument that records data	cardiograph
-graphy	the process of recording of data	cardiography
-ics	science or skill of	synthetics
-itis	red, inflamed, swollen	bursitis
-meter	means of measure	thermometer
-metry	action of measuring	telemetry
-ology/-ogy	the study of	biology
-phore	bearer or maker	semaphore
-phobia	intense, irrational fear	arachnophobia
-scope	instrument used for visualizing data	microscope
-scopy	visualize or examine	bronchoscopy

The following is a list of additional **medical terminology suffixes**:

Suffix	Meaning
-ac	pertaining to
-ad	toward
-al	pertaining to
-algia	pain
-apheresis	removal
-ar	pertaining to
-ary	pertaining to
-asthenia	weakness
-atresia	occlusion, closure
-capnia	carbon dioxide
-cele	hernia
-centesis	surgical puncture
-clasia	break
-clasis	break
-coccus	berry-like bacteria
-crit	separate
-cyte	cell
-desis	fusion
-drome	run
-eal	pertaining to
-ectasis	expansion
-ectomy	removal
-emia	blood dysfunction
-esis	condition
-gen	agent that causes
-genesis	cause
-genic	pertaining to
-ia	disease condition
-ial	pertaining to
-iasis	condition
-iatrist	physician
-iatry	specialty
-ician	a person skilled in
-ictal	attack
-ior	pertaining to
-ism	condition of
-lysis	separating
-malacia	softening
-megaly	increasing in size
-odynia	pain
-oid	resembling
-ologist	person that practices

Suffix	Meaning
-oma	tumor
-opia	vision
-opsy	view of
-orrhagia	blood flowing profusely
-orrhaphy	repairing
-orrhea	flow
-orrhexis	break
-osis	condition
-ostomy	to make an opening
-otomy	cut into
-ous	pertaining to
-oxia	oxygen
-paresis	partial paralysis
-pathy	disease
-penia	decrease in number
-pepsia	digestion
-pexy	suspension
-phagia	swallowing, eating
-phonia	sound, voice
-physis	growth
-plasia	development
-plasm	a growth
-plasty	repair by surgery
-plegia	paralysis
-pnea	breathing
-poiesis	formation
-ptosis	sagging
-salpinx	fallopian tube
-sarcoma	malignant tumor
-schisis	crack
-sclerosis	hardening
-sis	condition of
-spasm	abnormal muscle firing
-stasis	standing
-stenosis	narrowing
-thorax	chest
-tocia	labor, birth
-tome	cutting device
-tripsy	surgical crushing
-trophy	develop
-uria	urine

WORD ROOTS

The following is a list of common **medical terminology word roots**:

Root Word	Word	Root Word	Word
abdomin/o	abdomen	chrom/o	color
acou/o	hearing	clavic/o	clavicle
acr/o	height/extremities	col/o	colon
aden/o	gland	colp/o	vagina
adren/o	adrenal gland	core/o	pupil
alveol/o	alveolus	corne/o	cornea
amni/o	amnion	coron/o	heart
andro/o	male	cortic/o	cortex
angi/o	vessel	cor/o	pupil
ankly/o	stiff	cost/o	rib
anter/o	frontal	crani/o	cranium
an/o	anus	cry/o	cold
aponeur/o	aponeurosis	cutane/o	skin
appendic/o	appendix	cyan/o	blue
arche/o	beginning	cyes/I	pregnancy
arteri/o	artery	cyst/o	bladder
athero/o	fatty plaque	cyt/o	cell
atri/o	atrium	dacry/o	tear
auri/o	ear	derm/o	skin
aut/o	self	diaphragmat/o	diaphragm
azot/o	nitrogen	dipl/o	double
bacteri/o	bacteria	dips/o	thirst
balan/o	glans penis	disk/o	disk
bi/o	life	dist/o	distal
blast/o	developing cell	diverticul/o	diverticulum
blephar/o	eyelid	dors/o	back
bronchi/o	bronchus	duoden/o	duodenum
burs/o	bursa	dur/o	dura
calc/I	calcium	ech/o	sound
carcin/o	cancer	electr/o	electricity
cardi/o	heart	embry/o	embryo
carp/o	carpals	encephal/o	brain
caud/o	tail	endocrin/o	endocrine
cec/o	cecum	enter/o	intestine
celi/o	abdomen	epididym/o	epididymis
cephal/o	head	epiglott/o	epiglottis
cerebell/o	cerebellum	episi/o	vulva
cerebr/o	cerebrum	erythr/o	red
cervic/o	cervix	esophag/o	esophagus
cheil/o	lip	esthesi/o	sensation
cholangi/o	bile duct	eti/o	cause of disease
chol/e	gall	femor/o	femur
chondro/o	cartilage	feti/o	fetus
chori/o	chorion	fibr/o	fibrous tissue

Root Word	Word	Root Word	Word
fibul/o	fibula	mandibul/o	mandible
gangli/o	ganglion	mast/o	breast
gastr/o	stomach	maxill/o	maxilla
gingiv/o	gum	meat/o	opening
glomerul/o	glomerulus	melan/o	dark, black
gloss/o	tongue	mening/o	meninges
glyc/o	sugar	menisc/o	meniscus
gnos/o	knowledge	men/o	menstruation
gravid/o	pregnancy	ment/o	mind
gyn/o	woman	metri/o	uterus
hem/o	blood	mon/o	one
hepat/o	liver	muc/o	mucus
herni/o	hernia	myc/o	fungus
heter/o	other	myel/o	spinal cord
hidr/o	sweat	myelon/o	bone marrow
hist/o	tissue	myos/o	muscle
humer/o	humerus	nas/o	nose
hydr/o	water	nat/o	birth
hymen/o	hymen	necr/o	death
hyster/o	uterus	nephr/o	kidney
ile/o	ileum	neur/o	nerve
ili/o	ilium	noct/I	night
infer/o	inferior	ocul/o	eye
irid/o	iris	olig/o	few
ischi/o	ischium	omphal/o	navel
ischo/o	blockage	onc/o	tumor
jejun/o	jejunum	onych/o	nail
kal/I	potassium	oophor/o	ovary
kary/o	nucleus	ophthalm/o	eye
kerat/o	hard	opt/o	vision
kinesi/o	motion	orch/o	testicle
kyph/o	hump	organ/o	organ
lacrim/o	tear duct	or/o	mouth
lact/o	milk	orth/o	straight
lamin/o	lamina	oste/o	bone
lapar/o	abdomen	ot/o	ear
laryng/o	larynx	ox/I	oxygen
later/o	lateral	pachy/o	thick
lei/o	smooth	palat/o	palate
leuk/o	white	pancreat/o	pancreas
lingu/o	tongue	parathyroid/o	parathyroid gland
lip/o	fat	par/o	labor
lith/o	stone	patell/o	patella
lord/o	flexed forward	path/o	disease
lumb/o	lumbar	pelv/I	pelvis
lymph/o	lymph	perine/o	peritoneum
mamm/o	breast	petr/o	stone

47

Root Word	Word
phalang/o	pharynx
phas/o	speech
phleb/o	vein
phot/o	light
phren/o	mind
plasm/o	plasma
pleur/o	pleura
pneum/o	lung
poli/o	gray matter
polyp/o	small growth
poster/o	posterior
prim/I	first
proct/o	rectum
prostat/o	prostate gland
proxim/o	proximal
pseud/o	fake
psych/o	mind
pub/o	pubis
puerper/o	childbirth
pulmon/o	lung
pupill/o	pupil
pyel/o	renal pelvis
pylor/o	pylorus
py/o	pus
quadr/I	four
rachi/o	spinal
radic/o	nerve
radi/o	radius
rect/o	rectum
ren/o	kidney
retin/o	retina
rhabd/o	striated
rhin/o	nose
rhytid/o	wrinkles
rhiz/o	root, nerve
salping/o	tube
sacr/o	sacrum
scapul/o	scapula
scler/o	sclera
scoli/o	curved
seb/o	sebum
sept/o	septum
sial/o	saliva
sinus/o	sinus
somat/o	body
son/o	sound
spermat/o	sperm

Root Word	Word
sphygm/o	pulse
spir/o	breathe
splen/o	spleen
spondyl/o	vertebra
staped/o	stapes
staphyl/o	clusters
stern/o	sternum
steth/o	chest
stomat/o	mouth
strept/o	chain-like
super/o	superior
synovi/o	synovia
tars/o	tarsal
ten/o	tendon
test/o	testicle
therm/o	heat
thorac/o	thorax
thromb/o	clot
thym/o	thymus
thyr/o	thyroid gland
tibi/o	tibia
tom/o	cut
tonsil/o	tonsils
toxic/o	poison
trachel/o	trachea
trich/o	hair
tympan/o	eardrum
uln/o	ulna
ungu/o	nail
ureter/o	ureter
urethr/o	urethra
ur/o	urine
uter/o	uterus
uvul/o	uvula
vagin/o	vagina
valv/o	valve
vas/o	vessel
ven/o	vein
ventricul/o	ventricle
ventro/o	frontal
vertebr/o	vertebra
vesic/o	bladder
vesicul/o	seminal vesicles
viscer/o	internal organs
vulv/o	vulva
xanth/o	yellow
xer/o	dry

STANDARDIZED TERMINOLOGY AND ABBREVIATIONS

Standardized terminology and abbreviations are vital for patient safety. Use abbreviations to save time and space *only when there is no potential for confusion over the meaning of the message.* Avoid Latin if there is an accepted English equivalency. The Medical Records manager decides acceptable terminology and forbidden abbreviations. If you are working in a small office and in charge of Medical Records, use the list of safe terms from The American Society for Testing and Materials' (ASTM) and the list of dangerous abbreviations from the Institute for Safe Medication Practices (ISMP). The Joint Commission also has a "Do Not Use" List for medical abbreviations and symbols that are included on the ISMP's more comprehensive list. Post them throughout the office. Use one type of units only. For example, do not use SI units (International System of Measurement) for Lab and Imperial units for Pharmacy without listing equivalencies. Adopt the US Postal Service database's two-letter abbreviations for states.

Health professionals use abbreviations to save time when charting or to be discreet when speaking around a patient. Abbreviations take these **forms**:

- Brief form means shortening a common term or difficult to pronounce term, for example: "telephone" into "phone" and "Papanicolaou smear" into "Pap smear."
- Acronym means making a word out of a phrase, for example *laser* stands for light amplification by stimulated emission of radiation.
- Initialism means making a word from the first letters of words in a phrase, and pronouncing the series of letters, for example, MRI for magnetic resonance imaging or HIV for human immunodeficiency virus.
- Eponym means naming a test or sign for its discoverer, for example, Coomb's test and McBurney's sign.

Potentially lethal abbreviations to avoid are:

- **Homonyms**: Same pronunciation but different meaning, such as ileum and ilium.
- **Synonyms**: Different words with similar meanings, such as dead and deceased.

MEDICAL ABBREVIATIONS AND ACRONYMS

Abbreviation or Acronym	Meaning
AIDS	acquired immunodeficiency syndrome
A.D.	right ear, auris dextra (* on ISMP's list of error prone abbreviations)
A.S.	left ear, auris sinistra (* on ISMP's list of error prone abbreviations)
A.U.	both ears, auris utraque (* on ISMP's list of error prone abbreviations)
O.D.	right eye, oculus dexter (* on ISMP's list of error prone abbreviations)
O.S.	left eye, oculus sinister (* on ISMP's list of error prone abbreviations)
O.U.	both eyes, oculus uterque (* on ISMP's list of error prone abbreviations)
CA	cancer or carcinoma
CBC and diff	complete blood count and differential
CHF	congestive heart failure
TAHBSO	complete hysterectomy; total abdominal hysterectomy, bilateral salpingo-oophorectomy
CABG	(pronounced "cabbage") coronary artery bypass graft
DNR	do not resuscitate; no codes should be called for this patient and no heroic measures should be taken to revive patient if the patient stops breathing
DTR	deep tendon reflexes
D&C	dilatation and curettage, used to cure uterine bleeding or for early abortion
ECG or ECG	electrocardiogram
ELISA	enzyme-linked immunosorbent assay, used to test for antibodies and antigens
FABERE	flexion abduction external rotation extension test, part of a physical to measure the patient's range of motion
HPI	history of present illness
Laser	light amplification by stimulated emission of radiation, a tool to carve tissue
P&A	percussion and auscultation, as in, "The lungs were clear to P&A."
PVH	persistent viral hepatitis
PND	postnasal drainage (can also mean paroxysmal nocturnal dyspnea in a sleep study)
simkin	simulation kinetics analysis
p.c.	*post cibum*, after meals
a.c.	*ante cibum*, before meals
h.s.	*hora somni*, bedtime

ADDITIONAL COMMON ABBREVIATIONS

Abbreviation	Meaning
ad lib	Freely or whenever desired
ANS	Autonomic nervous system
ant	Anterior
ASAP	As soon as possible
AV	Arteriovenous
bid	Twice a day
BP	Blood pressure
bpm	Beats per minute
BUN	Blood urea nitrogen
Bx	Biopsy
C&S	Culture and sensitivity
Ca	Calcium
CC	Colony count
cc	Cubic centimeters
CEA	Carcinoma embryonic antigen
Cl	Chloride
cm	Centimeters
CNS	Central nervous system
CPK	Creatine phosphokinase
CPR	Cardiopulmonary resuscitation
CSF	Cerebrospinal fluid
CV	Cardiovascular
CVP	Central venous pressure
D/C	Discharge
DW	Distilled water
Dx	Diagnosis
EBL	Estimated blood loss
e.m.p.	In the manner prescribed
ERT	Estrogen replacement therapy
ESR	Erythrocyte sedimentation rate
etiol	Etiology
FBS	Fasting blood sugar
Fe	Iron
FSH	Follicle-stimulating hormone
g	Grams
GERD	Gastroesophageal reflux disease
Grad.	Gradually
GTT	Glucose tolerance test

Abbreviation	Meaning
gtt	Drops
hr	Hour
H or hypo.	Hypodermic
HD	Hemodialysis
H&H	Hemoglobin and hematocrit
Hct	Hematocrit
Hg	Mercury
Hgb	Hemoglobin
HIV	Human immunodeficiency virus
H&P	History and physical
IM	Intramuscular
IV	Intravenous
K	Potassium
KCl	Potassium Chloride
kg	Kilograms
KVO	Keep Vein Open
lab	Laboratory
meds	Medications
mEq	Milliequivalents
MS	Multiple Sclerosis
Na	Sodium
NB	Newborn
neg	Negative
NPO	Nothing by mouth
OD	Daily
O_2	Oxygen
PCV	Packed Cell Volume
PM	Between noon and midnight
pos.	Positive
post-op	Postoperatively
PRBC	Packed Red Blood Cells
p.r.n.	As needed
PSA	Prostatic specific antigen
PT	Prothrombin time
PT	Physical Therapy
qd	Every day
qid	Four times a day
qod	Every other day
q4h	Every four hours
stat	Immediately
tid	Three times a day

51

PLURALIZING MEDICAL TERMS

Most medical laboratory terms derive from Latin and Greek. Most Latinate terms originated from the Greek. The basic rules for pluralizing medical terms are as follows:

Rule	Example
a changes to –*ata*	Stigm*a* to stigm*ata* Condylom*a* to condylom*ata*
-*on* changes to -*a*	Criteri*on* to criteri*a* Phenomen*on* to phenomen*a*
-*s* changes to –*des*	Iri*s* to iri*des* Arthriti*s* to arthriti*des*
Feminine *a* ending changes to *ae*	Uln*a* to uln*ae* Conch*a* to conch*ae*
Masculine ending *us* changes to *i*	Radi*us* to radi*i* Muscul*us* to muscul*i*
Neuter ending *um* changes to *a*	Bacteri*um* to bacteri*a* Trepone*um* to Trepone*a*
-*osis* changes to -*oses*	Diagn*osis* to diagn*oses* Anastom*osis* to anastom*oses*
-*x* changes to –*ces* or –*ges*	Phalan*x* to phalan*ges* Vari*x* to vari*ces*

MEDICAL AND SURGICAL SPECIALTIES

The suffix -*ology* means "study of," and the suffixes -*iatry* and -*iatrics* refer to "medical treatment." Add the body system root to obtain the name of the specialty:

Term	Meaning
Anesthesiology	Study of pain relief
Bariatrics	Treatment of obesity
Cardiology	Study of the heart
Dermatology	Study of the skin
Endocrinology	Study of the hormone system
Gastroenterology	Study of the digestive system
Geriatrics	Treatment of the elderly
Hematology	Study of the blood
Neurology	Study of the nervous system
Obstetrics	Treatment of pregnant women
Pediatrics	Treatment of children
Psychiatry	Treatment of the mind
Radiology	Study of radiation (for medical imaging)
Rheumatology	Study of rheumatoid diseases, like arthritis
Toxicology	Study of poisons
Urology	Study of the urinary system

REFERENCE SOURCES FOR MEDICAL TERMINOLOGY

Reliable **reference sources** to check correct spelling, selection and use of medical terminology are listed below:

- **Abbreviations**: Use safe terms and definitions from The American Society for Testing and Materials (ASTM). Obtain a list of dangerous abbreviations to be avoided from the Institute for Safe Medication Practices (ISMP).
- **Style guides**: Provide guidelines for format and presentation in documents. Use the *American Medical Association Manual of Style: A Guide for Authors and Editors* for an overview.
- **Anatomy and physiology texts**: Contain essential information regarding body structure, function of body parts, disease processes, and common health disorders. *Grey's Anatomy* is the classic.
- **Specialty texts**: When help is required with specialty transcriptions, try Sloan's *Medical Word Book*, Tessier's *Surgical Word Book*, and Pagana's *Laboratory and Diagnostic Tests*.
- **English dictionary**: Helps with spelling, definitions, and pronunciation. *Cambridge Dictionary of American English* is the standard.

CONVERSION CHART OF METRIC TO ENGLISH

	Metric	**English**
Distance	meter	3.3 feet
Mass	gram	0.0022 pounds
	kilogram	2.2 pounds
Volume	liter	1.06 quarts

ROMAN NUMERALS

The following **Roman numerals** equal the Arabic numbers.

$$I = 1$$
$$V = 5$$
$$X = 10$$
$$L = 50$$
$$C = 100$$
$$D = 500$$
$$M = 1000$$

MILITARY AND CIVILIAN TIME

Military	=	Civilian	Military	=	Civilian
0100	=	1:00 AM	1300	=	1:00 PM
0200	=	2:00 AM	1400	=	2:00 PM
0300	=	3:00 AM	1500	=	3:00 PM
0400	=	4:00 AM	1600	=	4:00 PM
0500	=	5:00 AM	1700	=	5:00 PM
0600	=	6:00 AM	1800	=	6:00 PM
0700	=	7:00 AM	1900	=	7:00 PM
0800	=	8:00 AM	2000	=	8:00 PM
0900	=	9:00 AM	2100	=	9:00 PM
1000	=	10:00 AM	2200	=	10:00 PM
1100	=	11:00 AM	2300	=	11:00 PM
1200	=	12 Noon	0000	=	12 Midnight

FORMULAS AND CONVERSIONS

Fahrenheit into Celsius

$C = (F - 32) \times 5/9$

Celsius into Fahrenheit

$F = (C \times 9/5) + 32$

Pounds into kilograms

Kilograms = (Pounds × 0.4536)

Equation to determine percentage

(amount ÷ total) × 100 = percentage

APPROXIMATING LITERS OF BLOOD IN NORMAL ADULTS

The average adult has 70 mL of blood per kilogram of weight. In the United States, a person's weight is usually recorded in pounds. The phlebotomist will need to convert the pounds into kilograms by using the conversion factor of 0.4536. The person's weight in kilograms is multiplied by 70, the average mL of blood per kilogram. Then divide that number by 1000 to convert the mL into liters.

APPROXIMATING LITERS OF BLOOD IN INFANTS

The average infant has 100 mL of blood per kilogram of weight. If an infant's weight is given in pounds, it must be converted to kilograms using the conversion factor of 0.454. That number is then multiplied by 100, which is the average mL of blood per kilogram in an infant. Then divide that number by 1000 to convert the mL into liters.

Routine Blood Collections

Blood Sample Collection Supplies and Equipment

EQUIPMENT FOR BLOOD COLLECTION

Equipment needed for blood collection includes:

- Phlebotomy cart or tray to hold equipment for easy access.
- PPE, including gloves: Latex gloves should be avoided as many patients are allergic to latex, and powdered gloves pose a risk of sample contamination. Glove liners can be used for phlebotomists that are sensitive to gloves.
- Antiseptics: Isopropyl alcohol 70%, povidone iodine, and chlorhexidine gluconate are the most commonly used.
- Gauze pads and bandages: Cotton balls should not be used to apply pressure on the puncture site because they may adhere to the tissue and cause bleeding when removed.
- Vein-locating devices: Use if necessary and available.
- Tourniquet: Non-latex are preferable. Various sizes should be available, including extra-large for obese patients and pediatric sizes. They should be flat and about 1 inch in width. They may be disposable or reusable.
- Needles, syringes, tube holders, and evacuated collection tubes of various types, depending on the tests to be performed.
- Sharps container: These must be available to dispose of needles.

NEEDLE GAUGE AND SELECTION

The gauge of a needle is a number that is inversely correlates to the diameter of the internal space of the needle, for example, the larger the needle gauge the smaller the internal space of the needle and vice versa. Since color-coding varies between manufactures, be careful of relying on color to determine the gauge of a needle. When selecting a needle for venipuncture, there are several factors to consider which include the type of procedure, the condition and size of the patient's vein, and the equipment being used. The length of the needle used is determined by the depth of the vein. Keep in mind that the smaller the gauge the larger the bore. The 21-gauge needle is the standard needle used for routine venipuncture.

NEEDLE SAFETY DEVICES

Needle safety devices protect the needle user's hand by having it remain behind the needle during use and by providing a barrier between the user's hand and the needle after use. Also, needle safety devices are operable with a one-handed technique and provide a permanent barrier around the contaminated needle. By activating the safety device after use, the needle cover (generally a plastic top) clicks over the needle into a permanent, locked position. The needle cannot be reused nor inadvertently become exposed after the safety device is locked into place.

BUTTERFLY NEEDLE

If a patient, such as a child or adult who is very thin with prominent veins, requires a low needle angle or depth for venipuncture, the best choice is a **winged infusion ("Butterfly") set** that allows a very low angle (10-15°) for venipuncture as the needle can be held almost parallel to the skin. Winged needles are also useful to access hand veins and scalp veins of infants. The needle (usually 23-gauge, although 25-gauge may be used if vessels are extremely small) ranges from 0.5-0.75 inches in length with 6-15 inches of tubing to which the syringe is attached. Vacutainers can also attach to the end of the tubing on which blood collection tubes can be inserted and directly draw a sample. For insertion, the flexible wings are grasped to guide the needle. A flash can be observed in the collection chamber of the butterfly, and then blood withdrawn using the syringe or pressure of the vacutainer.

Butterfly Needle Infusion Set

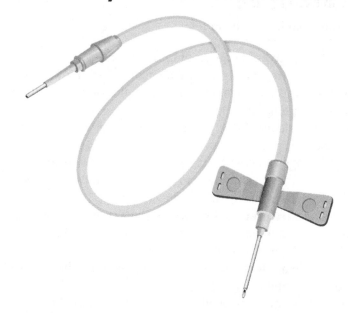

SYRINGE SYSTEM

In straightforward venipunctures, the syringe system may be used. A syringe is attached directly to the venipuncture needle that contains a small hub in which a "flash" can be visualized when the vein is accessed. The syringe can pull back the required volume of blood and then distribute that blood into the appropriate blood tubes.

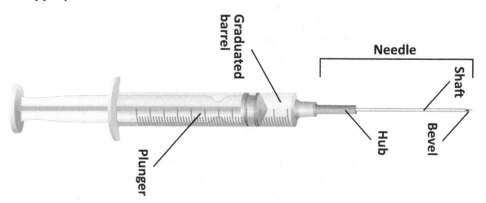

TOURNIQUET

A tourniquet is used to aid in the collection of a blood specimen. The tourniquet is tied in such a way that can be easily removed (using a quick release method) above the venipuncture site. The purpose of the tourniquet is to slow down venous flow away from the puncture site and to not inhibit arterial flow to the puncture site. By doing this, the vein enlarges to make it easier to locate and puncture. A tourniquet should not be left on longer than 1 minute because this may change the composition of the blood and make testing inaccurate.

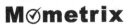

Blood Collection Additives and Collection Tubes

BLOOD COLLECTION ADDITIVES

ANTICOAGULANT

- EDTA
- Citrates
- Heparin
- Oxalates

ANTIGLYCOLYTIC AGENT

- Sodium fluoride
- Lithium iodoacetate
- Potassium oxalate

ADDITIVES FOUND WITH COLORED TUBE STOPPERS

- Yellow: ACD (acid-citrate-dextrose)
- Red (glass tube): No additive
- Light blue: Sodium citrate
- Lavender: EDTA
- Dark Green: Heparin
- Gray: Potassium oxalate and sodium fluoride
- Gold: silica, thixotropic gel
- Mottled red and gray: Silica, thixotropic gel

EDTA

Ethylenediaminetetraacetic acid (EDTA) is a potassium-based or sodium-based anticoagulant used in blood collection tubes (usually lavender and pink) to prevent clotting of the whole blood specimens (CBC and blood component tests) and to save specimens for blood bank testing. EDTA binds calcium to prevent clotting and preserves cell morphology and prevents the aggregation of platelets. The tube should be filled to the specified level and the correct tube size selected for the necessary volume. Eight to 10 inversions are needed immediately after sample collection in order to thoroughly mix EDTA with the blood because failure to adequately mix them can result in formation of microclots or aggregated platelets. EDTA may be in liquid form (K3EDTA) or spray-dried (K2EDTA), but the liquid form may dilute the sample and alter test results (1-2% decrease). EDTA tube with blood sample should be placed in a refrigerator while awaiting processing. The timing and storage requirements vary according to the type of test. For example, red blood cells count remains stable for up to 72 hours under refrigeration, but white blood cell counts are less stable.

HEPARIN

The purpose of heparin is to prevent coagulation. The three types of heparin are ammonium, sodium, and lithium. Ammonium heparin is used for hematocrit determinations and is found in capillary tubes. Sodium heparin and lithium heparin are used in evacuated tubes. Be sure that the heparin being used is not what is being tested. For example, heparin is used for electrolyte testing, but sodium is a commonly tested electrolyte, so sodium heparin would not be an appropriate heparin to use to test for electrolytes. It is important to mix heparin tubes properly to prevent microclots.

> **Review Video: Heparin – An Injectable Anti-Coagulant**
> Visit mometrix.com/academy and enter code: 127426

PPT, SST, AND PST

All three tubes contain thixotropic gel, which is a non-reactive synthetic substance that serves as an actual physical barrier between the serum and the cellular portion of a specimen after the specimen has been centrifuged. If thixotropic gel is used in a tube with EDTA, it is referred to as **a plasma preparation tube (PPT)**. When thixotropic gel is used in the serum collection tube, the gel is referred to as a serum separator, thus the tube and the gel are called the **serum separator tube (SST)**. When thixotropic gel is used in a tube with heparin, it is called a plasma separator. Thus, when thixotropic gel and heparin are in a tube, the tube is called the **plasma separator tube (PST)**.

COLLECTION TUBES BASED ON TEST

BLACK, DARK BLUE, AND LIGHT BLUE

Collection tube	Black	Blue (dark)	Blue (light)
Tests	ESR	Toxicology, trace metals, nutritional analysis	Coagulation
Additives	Sodium citrate	EDTA, heparin, or none	Sodium citrate
Specimen	Whole blood	Plasma or serum	Plasma
Inversions	0	Heparin or EDTA 8-10. No additive-0.	3-4
Department	Hematology	Hematology	Hematology
Notes	Do not invert. Fill tube completely.	Verify additive before proceeding.	Fill tube completely.

GOLD/TIGER-TOP/RED-GRAY, GRAY OR LIGHT GRAY, DARK GREEN

Collection tube	Gold, Tiger-top, Red-gray	Gray, Light gray	Green (dark)
Tests	Blood chemistries, serology, immunology	Lactic acid, GTT, FBS, blood alcohol	Blood chemistry, ammonia, electrolytes, ABG
Additives	Clot activator and/or thixotropic gel	Iodoacetate, sodium fluoride, and/or potassium oxalate or heparin or EDTA	Heparin (sodium)
Specimen	Serum	Plasma	Plasma or whole blood
Inversions	5-6	8-10	8-10
Department	Chemistry	Chemistry	Chemistry
Notes	AKA serum separator tube	May need to be placed on ice.	STAT test

LIGHT GREEN OR GRAY/GREEN, LAVENDER, AND ORANGE OR YELLOW-GRAY

Collection tube	Light green, Gray/green	Lavender	Orange, Yellow-gray
Tests	Potassium, chemistry tests	CBC, molecular tests	Chemistry tests
Additives	Heparin (lithium), thixotropic gel	EDTA	Thrombin
Specimen	Plasma	Whole blood	Serum
Inversions	8-10	8-10	8-10
Department	Chemistry	Hematology	Chemistry
Notes		Most common test	STAT test

PINK, RED (GLASS), RED (PLASTIC)

Collection tube	Pink	Red (glass)	Red (plastic)
Tests	Hematology, typing and screening	Chemistry, serology, immunology, crossmatch (for blood bank)	Chemistry, serology
Additives	EDTA	None	Clot activators
Specimen	Whole blood	Serum	Serum
Inversions	8-10	0	0
Department	Blood bank	Chemistry	Chemistry
Notes	Do not confuse pink and lavender tubes.	Specimen must rest 30 minutes. Do not confuse with plastic red tube.	Specimen must rest 30 minutes. Do not confuse with glass red tube.

TAN, STERILE YELLOW, NONSTERILE YELLOW

Collection tube	Tan	Yellow (sterile)	Yellow (nonsterile)
Tests	Lead analysis	Blood culture	HLA, paternity test, tissue typing
Additives	K2 or EDTA	SPS	Acid citrate dextrose (ACD)
Specimen	Plasma	Whole blood	Whole blood
Inversions	8-10	8-10	8-10
Department	Chemistry	Microbiology	Chemistry
Notes		Do not confuse with nonsterile yellow tube.	Do not confuse with sterile yellow tube.

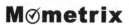

Blood Sample Collection Procedures

PRIORITIZATION OF SPECIMEN COLLECTION AND RESULTS

The nomenclature and scheme for the prioritization of specimen collection and results are as follows:

Priority	Discussion
1. STAT, Medical Emergency, Immediate	Patient critical or results needed immediately. Tests include glucose, cardiac enzymes, hemoglobin and hematocrit, and electrolytes. Collect sample immediately and alert laboratory technicians. STAT orders from ED usually have priority over inpatient STAT orders.
2. Timed specimen	Must be obtained as close to specified time as possible to ensure meaningful results. Tests include 2-hour PP GTT, cortisol, blood cultures, and cardiac enzymes. Note exact time of collection on sample.
3. ASAP (as soon as possible), Preop, and Postop	Patient is in serious but not critical condition. Tests include hemoglobin and hematocrit, electrolytes, and glucose. Preop is collected before surgery to verify suitability (CBC, platelet function, hemoglobin, hematocrit, PTT, and type and crossmatch) and postop to assess condition (hemoglobin, hematocrit). Some patients (preop) may be NPO.
4. Fasting	Verify fasting before collection. Tests include glucose, cholesterol, and triglycerides.
5. Routine	Collect when possible, but there is no urgency to do so because they are used to monitor condition or establish diagnosis. Tests include CBC and chemistry panels.

PROPER ANTISEPTIC AGENTS

Antiseptics inhibit organisms but do not kill all of them; however, the disinfectants that are better able to kill organisms are unsafe to use on skin. New CLSI recommendations stress the importance of cleaning the venipuncture site with friction as a means to destroy the most bacteria possible (rather than the classic concentric circle method previously recommended). A number of different antiseptics can be used for skin preparation for common phlebotomy tests:

- **Isopropyl alcohol 70%:** This is the most commonly used and recommended antiseptic as it is tolerated by most individuals and has good antiseptic qualities. It is usually supplied in individually wrapped pads.
- **Ethyl alcohol:** Generally, it needs to be a higher concentration and left on for a longer period of time than isopropyl alcohol.
- **Povidone-iodine/tincture of iodine:** Used when higher order antisepsis is needed, such as for blood cultures. However, many patients are allergic to iodine, so this limits use.
- **Benzalkonium chloride:** May be used as a substitute for alcohol, as indicated for when measuring blood alcohol levels.
- **Chlorhexidine gluconate:** Used when higher order antisepsis is needed, such as for blood cultures, and recommended for IV catheter sites. Must air dry completely to be fully effective.

VENIPUNCTURE PROCEDURES

LOCATING VEINS THAT ARE DIFFICULT TO VISUALIZE OR FEEL

When veins are difficult to visualize or feel, different techniques may be utilized:

- **Massage**: Gently massaging the arm starting at the wrist and moving proximally to the venipuncture site after applying the tourniquet may help veins stand out; however, excessive massaging may alter results.
- **Heat application**: Applying a heating pad or a warm moist compress to the site for 5 minutes may help to distend the vein by causing vasodilation, making the vein easier to locate.
- **Fist pumping**: After the tourniquet is applied, the patient should be asked to make a fist as this helps the veins to appear more prominent. However, repeatedly pumping the fist should be avoided because this may alter some test results (potassium, phosphate), and the movement may make the vein harder to locate.
- **Positioning**: Lowering the arm to a dependent position (such as over the side of the bed) may help to fill the veins and make them easier to locate. Rotating the arm may help to locate a vein.

> **Review Video: Starting and IV**
> Visit mometrix.com/academy and enter code: 380529

APPROPRIATE SITE FOR VENIPUNCTURE

The vein that is most commonly used for **venipuncture** is the median cubital, which joins the cephalic and basilic veins and is easily accessed in the antecubital space of the arm. Other veins that are sometimes used include the cephalic vein and the basilic vein. The basilic vein lies close to the median nerve and should, therefore, be the last choice. Additionally, the proximal portion of the vein lies near arteries, which can result in accidental arterial blood draw and excessive bleeding. The dorsal metacarpal veins in the hands are easily visible and accessible, but should usually be avoided in older adults because of little supporting subcutaneous tissue. The nerve most often injured with venipuncture is the median nerve because blood draws are most frequently done in the antecubital space, and the median nerve, which is the largest in the arm, passes through this area. The second most common injury is of the radial nerve, which runs near the cephalic vein on the radial side of the wrist and into the palm of the hand. A last resort vein would be the basilica vein because it rolls easily and is positioned so that the brachial artery and a major nerve are at risk for puncture if used. Ankle and foot veins should only be punctured at the discretion of a physician and should only be used when no other veins are appropriate. Poor circulation and clotting factors may affect results of tests and cause puncture wounds that may not readily heal. Venipuncture should be avoided in the 7.5 cm area above the thumb and on the palmar surface of the wrist.

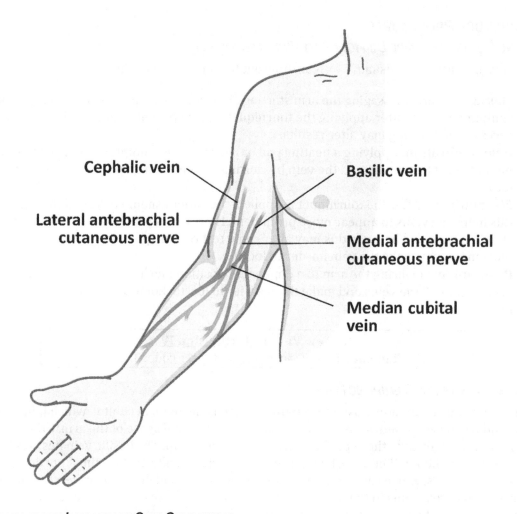

Cephalic vein

Basilic vein

Lateral antebrachial cutaneous nerve

Medial antebrachial cutaneous nerve

Median cubital vein

VARIABLES THAT INFLUENCE SITE SELECTION

The following are some variables that make a site **inappropriate** for selection:

1. Injuries to the skin such as burns, scars, and tattoos
2. Damaged veins from repeated collections or drug use
3. Swelling (edema)
4. Hematoma (bruising)
5. Mastectomy or cancer removal including skin cancer

SELECTING EQUIPMENT AFTER IDENTIFYING COLLECTION SITE

Selecting equipment after identifying the collection site allows the clinician to waste less equipment if the collection site turns out to be inappropriate for the equipment assembled. Also, this allows for adequate drying time for the alcohol (which is required for proper cleaning of the site and also reduces the sting from the alcohol). A site should have a minimum drying time of 30 seconds.

PERFORMING THE VENIPUNCTURE

The first step in blood collection after identifying the site, performing appropriate antisepsis, and gathering supplies is anchoring the vein. **Anchoring a vein** involves stretching the skin one inch below the site to provide a taut surface and securing the vein to minimize moving and rolling during puncture. When the puncture site is the antecubital area, the thumb should be placed one to two inches below the antecubital area pulling the tissue distally with the other fingers wrapped about the back of the arm to secure the arm. It's important to avoid a C-hold with the thumb below and index finger above the puncture site because this poses a risk of accidental needlestick if the patient jerks the arm way. If veins on the back of the hand are used, then the patient's hand should be grasped right below the knuckles, the patient's fingers bent, and the skin on the top of the hand stretched taut with the thumb. Most **needles** are inserted bevel up at an angle of 15-30°, depending on the vein depth, in a proximal direction. A slight decrease in resistance (often characterized as a "pop") is felt when the needle enters the vein.

VENIPUNCTURE IN SPECIAL POPULATIONS

PREFERRED METHOD OF RETRIEVING BLOOD FROM CHILD OR INFANT

Skin puncture is the preferred method for retrieving blood from a **child or infant** because children have smaller quantities of blood than adults which can lead to anemia if enough blood is drawn. Also, a child or infant may be hurt if they need to be restrained during a venipuncture. If a child moves around during venipuncture, it may result in an injury to nerves, veins, and arteries.

The first droplet of blood in a skin puncture contains excess tissue fluid, which may affect test results and should therefore be "wasted." Wasting will also allow the alcohol residue on the skin to be wiped away with the first droplet of blood. That alcohol can hemolyze the blood specimen and keep a round droplet of blood from forming. After wasting the first droplet, massaging around the site should generate a second droplet that should be collected for testing.

SAFEST PLACE FOR HEEL PUNCTURE IN INFANTS

NCCLS (National Committee for Clinical Laboratory Standards) states that the safest area for skin puncture in an infant is on the plantar surface of the heel, medial to the imaginary line extending from the middle of the big toe to the heel or lateral to an imaginary line extending from between the fourth and fifth toes to the heel.

Deep punctures of an infant's heel can lead to osteochondritis (inflammation of the bone and cartilage) and osteomyelitis (inflammation of the bone). Lancets that control the depth of the heel stick should be utilized when available to avoid this complication.

VENIPUNCTURE ON DIALYSIS PATIENTS

Dialysis patients often have an arteriovenous shunt or fistula (usually in the forearm) created for dialysis access to filter toxins from the blood. Neither the AV shunt nor the fistula should be used to draw blood, and any blood draw should be on the opposite side. Venipuncture should be minimized in order to save veins as shunts and fistulas usually have to be periodically replaced, so if patients have advanced kidney disease who may be candidates for dialysis or already have a shunt or fistula in place, the dorsal veins of the hands should be used for blood draws and the cephalic and antecubital veins avoided. Drawing blood from foot veins should be done only if no other access is available because of increased risk of complications. When possible, capillary blood should be used. If post-dialysis blood values for BUN, sodium, and calcium are ordered, blood should be drawn within 20 seconds to 2 minutes after discontinuation of dialysis to obtain accurate results. Plasma levels of BUN increase up to 20% within 30 minutes, so timing of the blood draw is critical.

63

ARTERIAL PUNCTURES
COMMON SITES FOR ARTERIAL PUNCTURE

The **radial artery is the preferred choice for arterial puncture**. It is located on the thumb site of the wrist and is most commonly used. The brachial artery is second choice. It is located in the medial anterior aspect of the antecubital area near the biceps tendon insertion. Femoral artery is only used by physicians and trained ER personnel. It is usually used in emergency situations or with patients with low cardiac output.

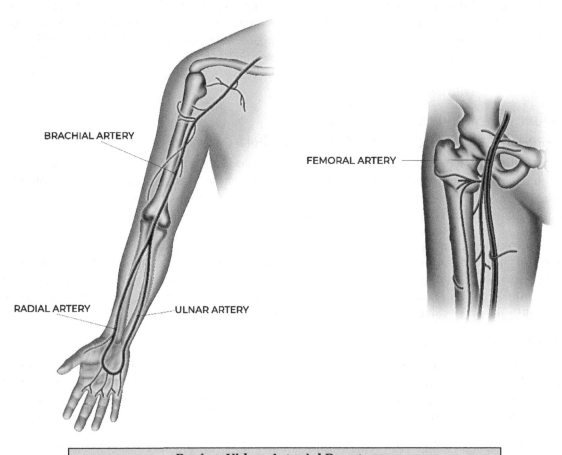

> **Review Video: Arterial Punctures**
> Visit mometrix.com/academy and enter code: 112543

ULNAR ARTERY AND THE ALLEN TEST

The purpose of the **Allen test** is to determine the presence of collateral circulation in the hand by the ulnar artery prior to an arterial puncture of the radial artery. The ulnar artery provides collateral circulation for the hand. Since the radial artery is most commonly used in arterial puncture, the ulnar artery is there as a back up to provide blood to the hand if the radial artery is damaged and becomes unable to supply blood to the hand. Ensuring the integrity of the ulnar artery is critical because if the radial artery is damaged and the ulnar artery is not providing sufficient blood flow, there is risk of serious damage to the hand.

The **Allen test** is as follows:

1. Compress the radial and ulnar arteries with fingers while the patient makes a fist.
2. Patient opens hand; it should have a blanched appearance.

3. The ulnar artery is released and the patient's hand should flush with color. If this occurs, the patient has a positive Allen test and has collateral circulation of the ulnar artery.

INVERSION

Inversion (the act of rotating a collection tube up and down) is carried out immediately after the blood sample is collected to mix an additive with the blood sample. Tubes without additives do not require inversions. Inversions must be done gently to thoroughly mix the additive with the sample. It's important to avoid shaking the tube or inverting too vigorously because this may result in hemolysis of the sample. If hemolysis occurs, then a number of different tests cannot be performed on the sample, including electrolyte and enzyme tests. If the inversions are done inadequately and the additive is not thoroughly mixed with the sample, microclots may develop, which could interfere with hematology tests. If inversion of gel separation tubes does not result in thorough mixing, this may interfere with clotting. The number of inversions needed varies according to the type of test and the type additive, but most additives require 8-10 inversions.

PREFERRED ORDER OF DRAW

Blood collection tubes must be drawn in a specific order to avoid cross-contamination of additives between tubes. The **recommended order** of draw is:

1. **Blood culture tube** (yellow-black stopper).
2. **Coagulation tube** (light blue stopper, sodium citrate additive). If a routine coagulation assay is the only test ordered, then a single light blue stopper tube may be drawn. If there is a concern regarding contamination by tissue fluids or thromboplastins, then one may draw a non-additive tube first, and then the light blue stopper. This sample must be filled completely to the fill line in order to be analyzed.
3. **Non-additive tube** (red stopper or SST).
4. **Additive tubes** in this order:
   a. Serum separator tube (SST, red-gray or gold stopper). Contains a gel separator and clot activator.
   b. Sodium heparin (dark green stopper).
   c. Plasma separator tube (PST, light green stopper). Contains lithium heparin anticoagulant and a gel separator.
   d. EDTA (lavender stopper).
   e. ACDA or ACDB (pale yellow stopper). Contains acid citrate dextrose.
   f. Oxalate/fluoride (light gray stopper).

POST CARE OF VENOUS, ARTERIAL, AND CAPILLARY PUNCTURE SITES

Post care for blood collection sites include:

- **Venous**: Place a folded gauze square over the puncture site, apply manual pressure for 1-2 minutes until bleeding stops (longer if necessary), and then cover with a pressure dressing or adhesive bandage.
- **Arterial**: Place a folded gauze square over the puncture site and apply manual pressure for 3-5 minutes (longer with anticoagulation or coagulopathy). If bleeding, swelling, or bruising persists after the initial period of manual pressure, continue pressure for an additional 2 minutes before checking again. The pressure should be maintained until all bleeding has stopped. A pressure bandage should never be used in lieu of manual pressure, and the patient should not apply pressure. Once bleeding stops, clean the area with povidone iodine or chlorhexidine and check again in two minutes. Check distal pulse. If unable to find a pulse after an arterial puncture or the pulse is faint, blood flow may be blocked partially or completely by a blood clot. Notify the patient's nurse or physician STAT so that circulation can begin to be restored as quickly as possible. Last, apply pressure dressing.
- **Capillary**: Apply pressure with a clean piece of gauze over the puncture site until bleeding stops. Because the puncture is so small, a bandage is not usually required but can be applied

Specific Blood Tests

BLOOD CULTURES

Blood collection for blood cultures usually involves collecting samples in two containers:

- **Aerobic container**: Contains air and a medium to encourage growth of aerobic organisms.
- **Anaerobic container**: A vacuum that contains no air but contains a medium to encourage growth of anaerobic organisms.

Blood cultures may be done to determine the cause of fever of unknown origin and to determine if bacteremia is present. If a needle and syringe is used to collect the specimen, the anaerobic container is filled first and then the aerobic container. If a winged infusion set ("butterfly") is used, then the aerobic bottle is filled first because the tubing may contain a small amount of air. If multiple sets are ordered at the same time, each set must either be obtained from a separate site, or by waiting 30 minutes between obtaining specimens (with fresh punctures for each collection). Blood culture specimens cannot be taken from preexisting peripheral or central intravenous catheters unless they are taken immediately upon the insertion of the IV.

BLOOD CULTURE PROCESS

The general blood culture collection process is as follows:

1. Verify patient identification with two identifiers.
2. Use standard precautions and venipuncture procedures, and use aseptic technique when handling equipment to avoid contamination.
3. Vigorously scrub skin with antiseptic (CHG is most widely recommended) for 30-60 seconds to remove skin bacteria and allow to dry.
4. Swab caps of blood culture bottles with antiseptic. Note fill line.
5. Carry out blood draw. Adults: 10-20 mL per set and pediatric patients 1-2 mL per set.
6. If multiple draws are ordered, wait 30 minutes between draws unless otherwise ordered. Take multiple draws from different sites if possible.
7. Replace venipuncture needle with blunt fill needle and use transfer device.
8. Inject blood culture specimen into both anaerobic and aerobic bottles.
9. Mix specimen with medium in the culture bottle according to directions.
10. Label culture bottles.
11. Dispose of contaminated equipment and sharps in appropriate containers.
12. Remove gloves, sanitize hands, and transport specimen to the laboratory. Incubate and monitor as per protocol.

TYPE AND ANTIBODY SCREEN OR CROSS-MATCH

Type and antibody screen or cross-match to determine blood type and compatibility may be performed for many reasons, while cross-matches are usually performed only for elective surgeries during which blood loss is probable. Type and screen (indirect Coombs test) identifies the blood type by identifying the A, B, and RH antigens and by screening for particular antibodies most commonly implicated in non-ABO hemolytic reactions. Type and screen is more often performed for procedures that result in <10% transfusions. Crossmatching (mixing donor and recipient blood to observe for agglutination) includes testing for immunoglobulin G antibodies and is performed if blood loss is probable. In emergencies, type-specific and partially cross-matched blood may be used, because this procedure takes less than 5 minutes. Otherwise, type-specific non-cross-matched blood is used, and as a last resort, type O-negative packed red blood cells are administered.

ETHANOL (BLOOD ALCOHOL) TEST

Ethanol (EtOH) tests, commonly referred to as blood alcohol tests, may be done for clinical or legal reasons. If carried out for legal reasons, such as to determine if a driver was under the influence of alcohol, chain-of-custody protocols must be followed and carefully documented. Special considerations include the following:

- Skin antiseptics containing alcohol (isopropyl alcohol, methanol, tincture of iodine) cannot be used because they may contaminate the specimen and alter test results. Alternative skin antiseptics include povidone-iodine and aqueous benzalkonium chloride. If no alternative is available, the site should be thoroughly washed with soap and water and dried.
- Alcohol readily evaporates, so the collection tube should be completely filled and the stopper should be left on the tube until ready to perform testing.
- Testing may be done on whole blood, serum, or plasma. A glass grey top, sodium fluoride tube, with or without anticoagulant, is usually used.

RED BLOOD CELLS

Red blood cells (RBCs or erythrocytes) are biconcave disks that contain **hemoglobin** (95% of mass), which carries oxygen throughout the body. The heme portion of the cell contains **iron**, which binds to the oxygen. RBCs live about 120 days after which they are destroyed and their hemoglobin is recycled or excreted.

The **morphology** of RBCs may vary depending upon the type of anemia:

- Size: Normocytes, microcytes, macrocytes.
- Shape: Spherocytes (round), poikilocytes (irregular), drepanocytes (sickled).
- Color (reflecting concentration of hemoglobin): Normochromic, hypochromic.

Hemoglobin measures the amount of oxygen-carrying hemoglobin protein in the blood, and **hematocrit** measures the percentage of RBCs in whole blood.

Collection and purpose are the same: Whole blood is collected in a lavender topped EDTA tube, microtainer (capillary tube), or from green-topped lithium or sodium-heparin tube. The sample should be inverted 6-8 times immediately after a blood draw. This test is done to assess anemia, hydration, polycythemia, and blood loss and to monitor therapy.

Normal Hemoglobin Values

- Varies by age/gender
  o Adult male: 13.2-17.3 g/dL
  o Adult female: 11.7-15.5 g/dL
- Critical values: <6.6 or >20 g/dL

Normal Hematocrit Values

- Varies by age/gender
  o Adult male: 38-51%
  o Adult female: 33-45%
- Critical values (Adults): <19.8% or >60%

Reticulocyte count: Measures marrow production and should rise with anemia. Normal values: 0.5-1.5% of total RBCs.

WBC Count and Differential

White blood cell (leukocyte) count is used as an indicator of bacterial and viral infection. **WBC count** is reported as the total number of all white blood cells.

- Normal WBC for adults: 4,800-10,000
- Acute infection: 10,000+
- Severe infection: 30,000
- Viral infection: 4,000 and below

The **differential** provides the percentage of each different type of leukocyte. An increase in the white blood cell count is usually related to an increase in one type, and often an increase in immature neutrophils (bands), referred to as a "shift to the left," is an indication of an infectious process:

- Normal immature neutrophils (bands): 1-3%. Increase with infection.
- Normal segmented neutrophils (segs) for adults: 50-62%. Increase with acute, localized, or systemic bacterial infections.
- Normal eosinophils: 0-3%. Decrease with stress and acute infection.
- Normal basophils: 0-1%. Decrease during acute stage of infection.
- Normal lymphocytes: 25-40%. Increase in some viral and bacterial infections.
- Normal monocytes: 3-7%. Increase during recovery stage of acute infection.

Normal Arterial Blood pH

pH is the measure of the acidity of a solution. pH is equal to the negative logarithm of the concentration of hydrogen ions in a solution. Generally speaking, a pH of 7 is neutral. Values less than 7 are considered acidic, and values greater than 7 are considered basic. A range of 6.5-7.5 is considered a neutral environment.

The normal range for **arterial blood pH** is 7.35-7.45. Acidosis is characterized by below normal blood pH. Alkalosis is characterized by above normal blood pH. This blood sample must be taken from an artery, as venous pH is not as accurate in assessing an individual's pH balance (although it is a secondary option of an arterial sample is not possible). Arterial samples can be collected using a straight stick, or by drawing off of an arterial line if the patient has this access.

ENDOCRINE SYSTEM BLOOD TESTS

Endocrine system blood tests include:

- **Aldosterone**: Aldosterone is a mineralocorticoid produced by adrenal glands in response to increased potassium, decreased sodium, or decreased blood volume. It helps to regulate sodium and potassium levels. Specimen is collected with plain red top tube and tested on serum (refrigerate after centrifugation). "Up-right" sample should be obtained after patient has been in a sitting position for at least 30 minutes.
- **Renin**: Renin is an enzymatic hormone secreted by the kidneys in response to sodium depletion. Tested to determine cause of hypertension. This test is usually conducted along with aldosterone level. The specimen is collected in a lavender-topped EDTA or pink-topped EDTA tube and is conducted on plasma.
- **Cortisol**: This is the primary glucocorticoid secreted by adrenal glands. It stimulates gluconeogenesis, serves as an insulin antagonist, suppresses inflammatory response, and mobilizes proteins and fats. This test assesses adrenal function and is used to diagnose Cushing's disease and Addison's disease. Specimen collected for the serum test is in the red or red/gray topped tube and specimen for plasma tests is in the green-topped heparin tube. If serial tests are required, the same type of tube should be used for all tests. Time of draw must be correctly noted. Tests are often done at 8 AM and 4 PM.
- **Glucagon**: This hormone is produced in the pancreas and excreted by kidneys, increasing the amount of glucose and fat in the blood. Specimen collected is in a chilled lavender-topped EDTA tube, and the test is conducted on plasma. Specimen must be tightly capped and placed in ice slurry for transport.
- **Insulin**: This hormone is produced in the beta cells of the pancreas, regulates metabolism of proteins, fats, and carbohydrates, and controls production and storage of glucose. This test is done to determine the amount of insulin secreted in response to glucose and may include the administration of a standardized dose of glucose at fixed time periods. The specimen is collected in a red-topped tube, and the test is conducted on serum.
- **Erythropoietin** (EPO): Hormone produced in the kidney promotes red cell production. This test assesses the cause of anemia and/or kidney function. The specimen is collected in a red, gold, or red/gray top tube, and the test is conducted on serum. Phlebotomy may increase levels of EPO.

COAGULATION TESTS AND PROCEDURE

Test [Normal range]	Procedure
Fibrinogen (factor I) [100-400 mg/dL]	Collect 1 mL blood in sodium citrate blue-capped tube (completely filled) for photo-optical clot detection. Synthesized in the liver, it converts to fibrin, which combines with platelets in coagulation sequence. Increased: acute MI, cancer, eclampsia, multiple myeloma, Hodgkin's disease, nephrotic syndrome, tissue trauma. Decreased: DIC, liver disease, congenital fibrinogen abnormality.
Fibrin degradation product (fibrin split products or FSPs) [<5 mcg/mL FEU*]	Collect 1 mL blood in sodium citrate blue-capped tube (completely filled) for latex agglutination test. Transport frozen. FSPs occur as clots form and more breakdown of fibrinogen and fibrin occurs, interfering with blood coagulation by coating platelets and disrupting thrombin, and attaching to fibrinogen so stable clots can't form. Increased: DIC, liver disease, MI, hemorrhage, pulmonary embolism, renal disease, obstetric complications, kidney transplant rejection.
Heparin assay (antithrombin III) [1-3 mo: 48-108% 1-5 yr: 82-139% 6-17 yr: 90-131% >18 yr: 80-120%]	Collect 1 mL blood in sodium citrate blue-capped tube (completely filled) for chromogenic immunoturbidimetry. Utilized to diagnose heparin resistance in patients receiving heparin therapy and to diagnose hypercoagulable conditions. Increased: Acute hepatitis, kidney transplantation, vit. K deficiency. Decreased: DIC, liver transplantation, nephrotic syndrome, pulmonary embolism, venous thrombosis, liver failure, cirrhosis, carcinoma.
Platelet aggregation [Results vary]	Collect 4-5 mL sample in sodium citrate tubes for analysis with light transmission aggregometer. Must be processed within 60 minutes of collection. Test measures the ability of platelets to aggregate and form clots in response to various activators. Decreased: Myeloproliferative disorders, autoimmune disorders, uremia, clotting disorders, and adverse effects of medications. Drugs that affect clotting should be avoided before a test for up to two weeks (on advice of physician).
Prothrombin time (PT) [10-14 seconds]	Collect 1 mL blood in sodium citrate blue-capped tube (completely filled). Increased: Anticoagulation therapy, vitamin K deficiency, decreased prothrombin, DIC, liver disease, and malignant neoplasm. Some drugs may shorten time. Critical value: >27 seconds.
Partial thromboplastin time (PTT) [60-70 seconds]	Collect 1 mL blood in sodium citrate blue-capped tube (completely filled). Increased: hemophilia A & B, von Willebrand's, vitamin deficiency, lupus, DIC, and liver disease. Critical value: >100 seconds.
Activated partial thromboplastin time (aPTT) [30-40 seconds]	Collect 1 mL blood in sodium citrate blue-capped tube (completely filled). Similar to PTT but an activator added that speeds clotting time. Used to monitor heparin dosage. Increased: Same as for PTT. Decreased: Extensive cancer, early DIC, and after acute hemorrhage. Critical value: >70 seconds.
D-Dimer [0.5 mcg/mL (measuring FEU*)]	Collect 1 mL blood in sodium citrate blue-capped tube (completely filled) for immunoturbidimetry. Transport frozen. D-dimer is a specific polymer that results when fibrin breaks down, giving a marker to indicate the degree of fibrinolysis. Increased: DIC, pulmonary embolism, DVT, late pregnancy, neoplastic disorder, preeclampsia, arterial/venous thrombosis.

FEU = fibrinogen equivalent units

C-REACTIVE PROTEIN AND ERYTHROCYTE SEDIMENTATION RATE

C-reactive protein is an acute-phase reactant produced by the liver in response to inflammation that causes neutrophils, granulocytes, and macrophages to secrete cytokines. Thus, levels of **C-reactive protein** rise when there is inflammation or infection. It has been found to be a helpful measure of response to treatment for pyoderma gangrenosum ulcers:

- Normal values: 2.6-7.6 μg/dL

Erythrocyte sedimentation rate (sed rate) measures the distance erythrocytes fall in a vertical tube of anticoagulated blood in one hour. Because fibrinogen, which increases in response to infection, slows the fall, the sed rate can be used as a non-specific test for inflammation when infection is suspected. The sed rate is sensitive to osteomyelitis and may be used to monitor treatment response. Values vary according to gender and age:

- <50: Males 0-15 mm/hr. Females 0-20 mm/hr.
- >50: Males 0-20 mm/hr. Females 0-30 mm/hr.

TRACE AND ULTRATRACE ELEMENTS

Trace elements are metals and may include iron, lead, zinc, mercury, aluminum, and copper. Ultratrace elements include boron, nickel, vanadium, arsenic, and silicon. Specimens may easily be contaminated so care must be taken to avoid any specimen containers with metal. Special trace-element-free specimen tubes (usually royal blue and containing EDTA, heparin, or no additive) should be used because trace metals may be found in standard glass and plastic tubes and in the stoppers. Because some substances—gadolinium, iodine, and barium contrast—interfere with test results, testing should be delayed for at least 96 hours if patients have received any of these. The specimens must be kept clean and protected from dust. No iodine products should be used for antisepsis, only alcohol. When transferring plasma or serum, it must be poured into aliquots and not transferred by a pipette. Labels are color-coded to indicate the type of additive: lavender indicates EDTA, green indicates heparin, and red indicates no additive.

BASAL STATE REQUIREMENTS FOR BLOOD TESTS

Some tests need to be carried out during a patient's **basal state**, which is the state the body is in when the patient awakes in the morning after 12 hours of fasting (no nutritional intake although water is usually allowed). In practice, patients are usually asked to fast for 8 to 12 hours, depending on the test. In addition to fasting, patients should be advised to avoid smoking, chewing any kind of gum, or exercising as these may alter the patient's basal state and affect test results. In some cases, patients may be asked to withhold alcohol or drugs for a period of time (often the day before the test). Tests that are usually done after fasting include:

- Glucose: 8 hours
- Triglycerides: 9-12 hours
- Lipids: 9-12 hours
- Renal function tests: 8-12 hours
- Vitamin B_{12} test: 6-8 hours
- Basic/comprehensive metabolic panels: 10-12 hours
- GGT: 8 hours
- Iron levels: 12 hours

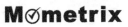

FACTORS INFLUENCING BASAL STATE

Factors that influence the basal state include the following:

- Age
- Altitude
- Daily variations
- Dehydration
- Diet
- Drugs (prescription and illegal)
- Exercise
- Fever
- Gender
- Humidity
- Jaundice
- Position
- Pregnancy
- Smoking
- Stress
- Temperature

Point of Care Tests

WAIVED TESTING

While laboratory testing is regulated by CLIA (Clinical Laboratory Improvement Amendments) and results are monitored through proficiency testing, some tests are considered to have a very low risk of error (although not necessarily error free), and the patient is unlikely to experience harm if a result is in error. These tests do not require proficiency testing. **Waived testing** includes specific tests exempted by CLIA regulations, tests approved by the FDA for home use (such as pregnancy tests), and tests for which the FDA has applied a waiver based on CLIA regulations and guidelines. Labs that carry out only waived testing must obtain a CLIA Certificate of Waiver (COW). Waived tests include dipstick or tablet reagent tests (such as for bilirubin and ketones), fecal-occult blood tests, blood glucose monitoring strips, ovulation tests (color-based), ESR tests, blood counts, and hemoglobin. Some states may require proficiency testing for tests that are waived under CLIA regulations, and some laboratories may choose to have proficiency testing of waived tests for internal quality control.

SPECIFIC POINT OF CARE TESTS

Point of care tests may give qualitative results (present or absent, such as pregnancy test) or quantitative result (precise numbers, such as glucose). Quality control is critical in ensuring that test results are accurate, and those performing the tests must be well-trained. Advantages include rapid turnaround time and small sample volumes. Additionally, a sample does not require pre-processing. Disadvantages include increased cost, quality variation, and billing concerns. Tests include:

- **Glucose**: A glucometer is used with a drop of blood from a finger obtained with a lancet and applied to a strip and inserted into the properly calibrated glucometer, which reports the results. Normal values for a child range from 60-100 mg/dL and for an adult under 100 mg/dL (fasting usually ranges from 70-100 mg/dL). Critical values are less than 40 g/dL or greater than 400 mg/dL. Non-glucose sugars, such as those in peritoneal dialysate, can affect results.
- **Coagulation**: Point-of-care tests for coagulation use a sample of whole blood to provide the patient's PT, aPTT, and INR for patients on warfarin anticoagulant. Some devices can measure activated clotting time (ACT) for patients on unfractionated heparin. For example, the CoaguChek X is a handheld meter used to monitor INR. A sample of capillary blood is obtained, and a drop of blood is placed on a test strip. The test strip must be inserted into the device within 15 seconds. Coagulation measurement begins, and the results are displayed. Test results for these devices are comparable to standard testing.
  - **INR**: (PT result/normal average): <2 for those not receiving anticoagulation and 2-3 for those receiving anticoagulation. Critical value: >3-5 in patients receiving anticoagulation therapy.
- **Pregnancy (human chorionic gonadotropin detection)**: Pregnancy tests are most accurate after a missed period and with the first morning urination. The patient should hold the testing stick in the stream of urine, or dip it in a cup of fresh urine. After the allotted wait time, the testing stick indicates whether the person is pregnant or not. False negatives may occur in early pregnancy.

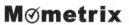

Phlebotomy Complications

ISSUES THAT AFFECT BLOOD COLLECTION

Various issues can affect the blood collection process and lead to complications. Many patients have allergies. These include possible allergies to adhesives, latex, and antiseptics. A patient may have a bleeding or bruising disorder that results from a genetic reason or medication that they are taking. Some patients may faint (syncope) during a procedure. It is very appropriate to recline a patient or have them lay down if they have fainted before. Some patients have a fear of needles. Some may experience nausea and vomiting from fear or an illness they have. It may be necessary to have a trash can or spit-up container nearby for easy access. If a patient is overweight or obese collection may be difficult.

VASOVAGAL REACTION

A vasovagal reaction, characterized by hypotension, diaphoresis, syncope, and nausea, may occur when a patient receives a venipuncture. If a patient complains of feeling faint and appears suddenly pale and shaky during a venipuncture (a vasovagal reaction characterized by diaphoresis and hypotension) the initial response should be to remove the needle because if the patient faints and falls the needle could be dislodged, resulting in trauma. As soon as the needle is removed, sitting patients should be assisted to put their heads low, between their legs. However, the patient is at risk of a fall injury, so the phlebotomist must support the patient. If the patient is in bed, the head of the bed should be lowered. If the patient faints and falls, an incident report must be completed and the patient examined and treated for any injury. The patient may need time to recuperate before another venipuncture is attempted.

NAUSEA AND VOMITING

Patients may experience nausea and vomiting before, during, or after venipuncture because of a nervous response, vasovagal reaction, or current illness. If a patient complains of nausea before the venipuncture begins, the phlebotomist should wait until the symptoms subside unless it is an emergent situation. An emesis basin should be provided for the patient, and the patient should be encouraged to take slow deep breaths to help the person relax. In some cases, applying a cold damp cloth to the patient's forehead may help. If the patient begins to vomit during venipuncture, the procedure should be stopped immediately, and a nurse should be called to assist the patient. The patient should be offered tissues to wipe the mouth and water to rinse the mouth (unless NPO). Some tests may induce nausea in patients, such as the glucose tolerance test.

COMPLICATIONS IN PATIENTS WITH CLOTTING DEFICIENCIES

Patients with clotting deficiencies or on anticoagulant therapy, such as warfarin or heparin, may **bleed excessively** after venipuncture. Patients are especially at risk for hematomas and persistent bleeding after venipuncture. Steady and prolonged pressure must be applied until bleeding stops. Elevating the arm may help to slow bleeding. A pressure dressing should not be placed instead of maintaining pressure until bleeding stops completely although a pressure dressing may then be applied and left in place for 20-30 minutes after bleeding stops as a precaution. Care must be taken to avoid excessive pressure, which may increase bruising. The phlebotomist should be aware that stroke and heart patients (such as those with atrial fibrillation) often take anticoagulants and should question medications. **Petechiae** may be a sign that a patient has a clotting deficiency, so the phlebotomist should examine the patient's skin carefully and be alert for excessive bleeding after venipuncture.

HEMATOMA

During a venipuncture, if the needle goes through the vein and a **hematoma** begins to rapidly develop, the next step is to remove the needle and tourniquet and apply pressure to prevent further loss of blood into the tissue. A hematoma may also form if the needle only partially penetrates the vessel wall, allowing blood to leak into the tissue. If blood flow stops and a small hematoma begins to form, the needle's bevel may be up against a vessel wall, so rotating it slightly may stop the leak and allow blood to flow into the collection tube. If a very small hematoma is evident during venipuncture, the best initial response is to observe the site and complete the venipuncture. If, however, the hematoma is large or expanding, then the phlebotomist should remove the needle, elevate the arm above the level of the heart, and apply pressure until the bleeding stops. Small hematomas are fairly common, especially in older adults whose veins may be friable and those taking anticoagulants and certain other drugs.

HEMATOMA CAUSES

Hematomas most often result from the following:

- Inadequate pressure to the collection site after a blood draw
- Blood leaking through the back of a vein that was pierced
- Blood leaking from a partially pierced vein
- An artery that was pierced

NERVE INJURY AND SEIZURES

Nerve injury can occur when the needle touches a nerve during a venipuncture, usually the result of poor site selection, improper insertion of needle, or patient movement. The pain is acute, and the patient will generally call out and complain of severe pain, tingling, or "electric shock." The phlebotomist must immediately remove the needle to prevent further damage. Once the bleeding is controlled, an ice pack applied to the site may help to decrease inflammation and pain. The phlebotomist must fill out an incident report and must follow procedures in accordance with facility protocols. Pain may persist for an extended period, and some patients may require physical therapy if nerve damage is severe.

Seizures are an uncommon complication and generally unrelated to venipuncture; however, if a seizure occurs, the phlebotomist should immediately discontinue the venipuncture, apply pressure to the insertion site without restraining the patient and call for help. The phlebotomist should try to prevent the patient from harm. If the patient is seated, the patient may need to be eased onto the floor with assistance. Place the patient side-lying on their left side if possible.

EDEMA AND PRIOR MASTECTOMY

Blood should not be drawn from edematous tissue because the **edema** may result in the blood diluted with tissue fluids. Edema is often most pronounced in the hands and feet, but arms may be edematous as well. With generalized edema, the phlebotomist should try to find the least edematous site for venipuncture, should apply gentle pressure to the site to displace the fluid if possible, and should note on the label that edema was present.

Blood generally should not be obtained on the side of a **mastectomy**, regardless of the length of time since surgery, because the circulation may be impaired, and edema may be present. Any degree of lymphedema may alter the results of the blood tests, and the patient is at increased risk of infection from venipuncture. If no other site is available, then a physician's order should be obtained regarding use of this site. With a double mastectomy, especially if any degree of lymphedema is evident, alternate sites, such as feet and legs may need to be considered. If possible, a sample may be obtained through capillary puncture for lymphedema, but for generalized edema, the sample will be diluted.

PRE-EXISTING INTRAVENOUS LINE

Blood samples should not be obtained from an **existing intravenous line** because the sample may be contaminated with IV fluids/drugs or diluted. Additionally, the sample is more likely to undergo hemolysis and need to be discarded.

Blood should also not be drawn from the same side as an IV line if possible. If blood must be drawn from an arm that has an intravenous line in place, the IV should be clamped for at least two minutes before the specimen is collected to allow the IV fluid to enter the circulation and reduce the dilution of the blood sample. It is preferable to do the venipuncture at least 5 inches distal to the IV insertion site when possible, with the tourniquet also applied distal to the IV insertion site. The site (proximal or distal) in relation to the IV should be documented.

ALLERGIES

Patients should be questioned about allergies prior to having blood withdrawn. **Common allergies** that may pose a problem include:

- **Latex**: Reactions range from mild to severe anaphylaxis, and latex allergies are increasingly common for those with frequent contact with healthcare, especially those with multiple surgeries and those with spina bifida. The phlebotomist should avoid taking any latex items, such as tourniquets and bandaging supplies, near the patient with a severe allergy and should generally replace latex items with non-latex for all patients.
- **Iodine**: Patients may be allergic to any skin antiseptic, but allergy to iodine is most common. Patients who report being allergic to fish are also at risk for iodine allergy. Alternate antiseptics should be used in place of antiseptics with iodine.
- **Adhesive**: Some patients are allergic to adhesive, which may cause itching and rash. Some types of tape, such as paper tape, are better tolerated but may still cause a problem for some patients. Stretch bandaging materials (such as Coban) may be used to secure a dressing.

MEDICATIONS AND RECENT SURGERY

Medications that pose a particular concern with phlebotomy are those that interfere with clotting mechanisms:

- **Platelet inhibitors**, such as aspirin and clopidogrel (Plavix).
- **Anticoagulants** including injectable drugs such as heparin, argatroban, and bivalirudin and oral anticoagulants, such as warfarin (Coumadin), rivaroxaban (Xarelto) and dabigatran (Pradaxa).

All of these drugs increase the risk of bleeding, so multiple venipunctures should be avoided when possible. Care must be taken to apply pressure until all bleeding stops, and a compression dressing may then be left in place for at least 20 minutes to ensure no recurrence of bleeding.

Recent surgery may pose a risk of complications, depending on the type of surgery and the medications given to the patient after surgery. Blood should not be drawn from an arm that has recently undergone any type of surgical procedure or the arm on the side of a mastectomy or any surgery that might interfere with blood flow or lymph flow.

DEHYDRATION AND CHEMOTHERAPY

Dehydration may occur in patients with severe nausea and vomiting and/or diarrhea and those with inadequate fluid intake for body needs. **Dehydration** results in decreased cardiac output and blood volume, so blood vessels constrict, making it difficult to access the veins and resulting in hemoconcentration that affects test results. If possible, the blood draw should be delayed until the patient is more hydrated, but if it is necessary to draw blood, a warm compress may help to dilate the vessels slightly. A smaller gauge needle or a winged infusion set may also be necessary. The label should indicate the patient is dehydrated and the physician notified.

Patients on **chemotherapy** often have central lines, such as ports or PICC lines and these may, at times, be used to withdraw samples, but phlebotomists are generally prohibited from drawing specimens through central lines. Veins may be fragile and collapse easily, so a smaller gauge needle or winged infusion set may be necessary. Warming the site may help to make the veins more visible. Edema may obscure veins, and prolonged bleeding may occur because of coagulopathy.

GERIATRICS

Drawing blood from geriatric patients poses a number of challenges:

- **Disabilities**: Patients may be hard of hearing and/or have difficulty speaking, interfering with communication with the patient. The phlebotomist should speak clearly without shouting and allow the patient extra time to respond or indicate comprehension. For patients with vision impairment, the phlebotomist should guide the patient and explain all actions verbally. If a patient has dementia, the phlebotomist should speak in simple sentences and reassure the patient, asking for help if the patient is hostile or combative. Physical disabilities (arthritis, neuromuscular diseases, contractures) may limit mobility.
- **Aging**: Loose skin and loss of muscle tissue may make it difficult to anchor a vein, and veins may be sclerosed or rolling, so careful anchoring of the vein is necessary. Scarred, sclerosed veins should be avoided. Circulation may be impaired (especially with diabetic patients), and medications (such as anticoagulants) may increase bleeding or interfere with test results. Prolonged pressure may need to be applied to puncture sites, and heavy adhesives may tear skin.

OBESITY

Obesity can pose a problem for venipuncture because the patient's veins may be deep and not visible or palpable. The median cubital vein in the antecubital area should be examined first as it may be palpable between folds of tissue. However, with obese patients, the cephalic vein is often easier to palpate than the median cubital vein. Rotating the hand into prone position (palm down) may make the cephalic vein more palpable. In some cases, a longer needle may be necessary for venipuncture. If there is no or little fat pad on the top of the hand, then the hand veins may be used for venipuncture. Tourniquets may be difficult to position as they tend to roll and twist. An extra-large tourniquet or Velcro closure strap should be used if possible but, if not available, using two tourniquets, one on top of the other, may help keep the tourniquet from twisting. Patients may know from past experience which access site is best, so the phlebotomist should ask the patient directly.

Special Collections

COLLECTION AND PRESERVATION OF EXTRAVASCULAR BODY FLUIDS FOR CHEMICAL ANALYSIS

Collection and preservation procedures for the chemical analysis of extravascular body fluids is dependent on fluid type.

Amniotic fluid	Sample is collected by a physician during amniocentesis. Store in a special container (protected from light) at room temperature for chromosome analysis or on ice for some chemistry tests (according to protocol).
Cerebrospinal fluid	Sample is collected by a physician. Collect in 3 tubes (first for culture and others for chemistry and microscopy) and store at room temperature with immediate delivery to lab. *Neisseria meningitidis* is fragile and cold sensitive, so do not chill the specimen.
Gastric fluids	Sample is collected during gastroscopy or from NG tube. Store in a sterile container at room temperature for up to 6 hours, refrigerated for up to 7 days, and frozen for up to 30 days.
Nasopharyngeal secretions	Collected with swab from nasopharyngeal area. Place swab in tube with transport medium.
Saliva	Collected in sterile container after the patient rinses mouth and waits a few minutes. Test immediately (point of care) or freeze for hormone tests to maintain stability.
Semen	Collect fresh sample from individual immediately following ejaculation into sterile container. Keep the sample warm and deliver immediately for testing.
Serous fluid	Sample is collected by a physician, typically through thoracentesis or paracentesis. Samples are labeled as pleural, peritoneal, or pericardial. Place in a sterile container for C&S, EDTA tube for cell counts/smears, and oxalate or fluoride tubes for chemistry tests.
Synovial fluid	Sample is collected by a physician through aspiration of the joint. Place in ETDA or heparin tube for cell counts, smear, and crystal identification; sterile tube for C&S; and plain tube for chemistry and immunology tests.
Sputum	First morning production of sputum preferred because a larger volume is likely to be produced after sleeping. Patients should remove any dentures and rinse mouth before attempting to cough up specimen. Transport at room temperature and process immediately.
Urine	Collected in sterile container form midstream urination or catheterization. If for 24-hour quantitative testing, urine is collected in a 2L container. Store at room temperature in sterile container for 2 hours (protected from light) and then refrigerate. If both UA and C&S required, then test or refrigerate immediately.

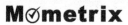

OROPHARYNGEAL AND NASOPHARYNGEAL SWABS

When obtaining an oropharyngeal or nasopharyngeal swab, the first steps are to wash the hands and don personal protective equipment, including gloves, a mask, and goggles (especially important if the patient is coughing). Seat the patient upright or with the head of the bed elevated to at least 45° and the head tipped back (pillows behind shoulders):

- **Oropharyngeal**: Depress the anterior third of tongue with tongue blade and insert swab without touching the lips, teeth, inside of cheeks, or tongue. Swab both tonsillar areas, moving the swab side to side (including any inflamed areas), and carefully remove the swab, avoiding contact with other tissues. Insert into sterile collection tube, break off stick, secure, and label.
- **Nasopharyngeal**: After the patient blows the nose, ask the patient to occlude one nostril at a time and exhale through the nose to determine if nostrils are clear. Carefully insert the swab through the nose (or nasal speculum if necessary) to the inflamed tissue, rotate the swab in the tissue, and remove the swab without touching other nasal tissue or the speculum. Save as above.

COLLECTION OF STOOL SPECIMENS

Stool specimens are obtained by placing a stool collection device in a toilet or in a bedpan. The specimen is then placed in a clean specimen container, or if for cultures, in a sterile container. Different types of containers may be used, with or without preservatives, depending on the type of tests being conducted. The sample is transferred using a tongue depressor to the fill-line indicated on the container. If an additive is in the container, the sample should be shaken to mix contents. The container should be properly labeled and sealed in a biohazard bag for transport. For a stool culture, the specimen should be collected before the patient begins antibiotics. The stool specimen is placed in a sterile container or a cotton-tipped swab is inserted into the rectum and rotated to obtain a fecal sample. Then the swab is inserted into a sterile tube. Stool specimens should be processed as soon as possible or stored at 4° C if there will be a delay of more than two hours before processing.

AFP

AFP is **alpha-fetoprotein**. Normally it is found in the human fetus, but abnormal levels of AFP may indicate a neural tube defect in an infant or other fetal developmental problems. The test is performed on maternal serum. If results are abnormal, a test on the amniotic fluid will be used to confirm results.

URINE TESTS

The following are some common urine tests:

- Routine urinalysis
- Culture and sensitivity: Diagnosis urinary tract infection
- Cytology studies: Detects presence of abnormal cells from urinary tract
- Drug screening: Detects use of illegal drugs (prescription or illicit) and steroids, and monitors therapeutic drug use
- Pregnancy test: Confirms pregnancy by testing for the presence of HCG

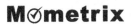

ASPECTS OF URINE REVIEWED IN ROUTINE URINALYSIS

The following are aspects of urine that are reviewed in a routine urinalysis:

- **Physical**: Color, odor, transparency, specific gravity
- **Chemical**: Looking for bacteria, blood, WBC, protein, and glucose
- **Microscopic**: Urine components (i.e., casts, cells, and crystals)

MIDSTREAM URINE COLLECTION AND MIDSTREAM CLEAN-CATCH URINE COLLECTION

Both the midstream urine collection and the midstream clean-catch urine collection methods involve an initial void into the toilet, interruption of urine flow, restart of urination into a collection container, collection of a sufficient amount of specimen, and voiding of excess urine down the toilet. The clean-catch involves cleaning of the genital area, collecting urine into a sterile container and quickly processing it to prevent overgrowth of microorganisms, degradation of the specimen, and incorrect results.

24-HOUR URINE SPECIMEN COLLECTION

For the 24-hour urine specimen test, all of the patient's urine must be over the course of **24 hours**. A large collection container is provided to the patient. When a patient awakes, the first void of the morning is for the previous 24 hours and must be discarded. The next void is collected as well as all additional voids over the next 24 hours (including the next morning's void). This specimen collection **must be kept cold**, and therefore mut be refrigerated or kept on ice during the 24-hours of collection.

Processing

SPECIMEN HANDLING AND TRANSPORTING
CHAIN-OF-CUSTODY SPECIMENS

Chain-of-custody specimens are those for which a laboratory has established a documented record that shows every consecutive person in contact with the specimen from the time of collection through transfer and to the time of disposition (both internal and external contact and including date, time, and signature) and ensures that no tampering with the specimen has occurred in order to meet legal requirements. The document must outline provisions for securing long-term storage. Chain-of-custody specimens may include specimens for blood alcohol, drugs, or crime scene testing, often including blood, urine, and DNA testing. The chain-of-custody SOP may include labeling requirements, temperature requirements, expected timeline, packing, and transporting specifications. The person from whom the sample is obtained must be clearly identified as well as the name of the collector and the time, date, and location of obtaining the sample. Containers in which a sample is transported should be secured with custody tape.

SPECIMEN ASSESSMENT AND REJECTION CRITERIA

Specimens must be obtained following established protocols and in the proper tube or container with the correct additive, such as sodium citrate in a blood specimen. The specimen must be stored and/or transported in a manner appropriate to the type of specimen. **Rejection criteria** may vary according to the type of specimen and test, and specimens are generally not discarded until the ordering healthcare provider is notified. Rejection criteria may include:

- Incorrect tube or container
- Incorrect or missing requisition/order
- Specimen size insufficient for testing
- Hemolysis evident
- Specimen not correctly labeled
- Tube/container leaking or contaminated with body fluids. (Note: critical specimens may be salvaged after the tube/container is thoroughly cleansed with 10% hypochlorite [bleach] solution.)
- Specimen contained in syringe with attached needle
- Date/collection time not noted on specimen
- Specimen too old for testing
- Specimen improperly stored/transported

ISSUES OF SPECIMEN QUALITY

Issues of specimen quality include:

- **Hemolysis**: Pink discoloration of plasma and serum because of the presence of damaged red blood cells and hemoglobin. May result from an abnormal condition, such as hemolytic anemia, or from incorrect handling. Hemolyzed samples may interfere with some tests (electrolytes, iron, enzymes), so the sample will likely need to be redrawn.
- **Quantity not sufficient (QNS)**: May occur if the volume of blood in the collection tube is insufficient for testing or if the blood-anticoagulant ratio is incorrect. Short draws may be sufficient for some tests if the specimen is not hemolyzed. With QNS, the usual solution is to obtain another specimen.
- **Clotting**: May result from maintaining a sample in a syringe with no anticoagulant for too long before transferring to a tube, carrying out a very slow draw with a syringe that allows clotting to begin, and failing to adequately mix the sample with the anticoagulant. If clotting occurs, a new sample must be obtained.
- **Incorrect specimen type**: If the incorrect specimen type is obtained or a specimen is obtained in a collection tube with the wrong additive, then a new specimen must be obtained in order to carry out the intended tests.

PROCEDURES TO PREVENT HEMOLYSIS

Hemolysis, rupture of red blood cells, is the most common reason laboratory specimens must be redrawn. Methods to prevent hemolysis include:

- Utilize large gauge (20-22) needle for blood draws for large veins, such as the antecubital.
- Warm the draw site to improve blood flow.
- Keep the tourniquet on for no longer than 60 seconds.
- Air-dry alcohol applied to skin prior to blood draw.
- Utilize partial vacuum tubes if possible.
- Avoid milking veins or capillary puncture sites.
- Avoid excessive pressure when pulling or pushing on the plunger.
- Avoid blood draws from catheters or vascular access devices.
- Ensure volume in tubes with anticoagulant is sufficient.
- Avoid vigorous mixing or shaking of specimens.
- Invert tubes with clot activator 5 times, with anticoagulant 8-10 times, and with sodium citrate 3-4 times (coagulation tests).
- Store and transport specimens at appropriate temperature.
- Use appropriate centrifugal speed and duration for processing samples that have clotted completely.

CLOTTING TIME CONSIDERATIONS FOR BLOOD SAMPLES

Clotting time may vary according to environmental conditions and addition of clot activators. Clotting must be fully complete before a sample is placed in the centrifuge or a latent formation of fibrin may clot serum. Complete clotting usually takes 30-60 minutes at temperatures of 22-25 °C (room temperature) although this time may be prolonged in samples with a high white blood cell count or in chilled samples. Clotting is also prolonged in samples of patients on anticoagulant therapy, such as heparin or warfarin. Clot activators may be added to a sample to decrease the time needed for clotting:

- Silica particles (found in serum separator tubes) and plastic red-topped tubes require 15-30 minutes.
- Thrombin tubes require about 5 minutes.

Note: 5-6 gentle inversions of tubes with clot activators to mix it with the blood sample are required.

SHIPPING PATIENT SAMPLES

The personnel responsible for shipping specimens must have been appropriately trained and understand possible hazards, according to regulations by the Department of Transportation, International Civil Aviation Organization, and CDC. Frozen serum and plasma must be shipped in plastic tubes (not glass) with screw-on caps for security and labeled with 2 patient identifiers. The tubes are wrapped in absorbent material in case of leakage, secured in a container that is airtight (such as Saf-T-Pak®), labeled "biohazard," and placed inside of a Styrofoam container for insulation with dry ice and in a clearly labeled secure box or in a temperature-controlled container. Specimens that are not frozen are similarly packaged using a specimen container, wrapped in absorbent material, placed in individual biohazard bags, and secured in transport box of metal or plastic. The specimen may or may not be placed in a temperature-controlled container, depending on ambient temperatures.

LIGHT CONSIDERATIONS IN TRANSPORTING SPECIMENS AND DISPOSITION OF SPECIMENS

Most specimens are not sensitive to **light**, but some must be transported in special light-blocking containers or wrapped in aluminum foil during transport: bilirubin, carotene, red cell folate, serum folate, vitamin B_2, 6, and 12, and vitamin C. Urine specimens for porphyrins and porphobilinogen must also be protected from light. Light-blocking amber colored collection tubes and urine specimen containers are also available. OSHA and state regulations outline the requirements for **disposition** of blood bags and patient samples. Blood disposition must comply with OSHA's Bloodborne Pathogen's Standard (29 CFR 1910.1030), which covers blood (semi-liquid, liquid, dried) in containers, in other waste products, or on items, such as sharps. As a regulated waste, the blood must be placed in a container that is closable, leak-proof, labeled (proper color-coding), and closed before removal to avoid any spillage or loss of contents during transport to disposal site.

SPECIMEN PROCESSING
PROPERLY CENTRIFUGING A SPECIMEN

The centrifuge needs to be evenly balanced with tubes of equal size and volume across from one another. Stoppers should always be in place to prevent aerosol. Also, be sure to allow complete clotting before centrifuging the specimen. If a specimen is not completely clotted before centrifuging it may result in latent fibrin formations clotting the serum. Never centrifuge a specimen twice.

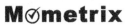

SETTLING OF BLOOD IN ANTICOAGULANT TUBES

Blood in an anticoagulant tube will settle in this manner after being centrifuged or allowed to settle:

- The top layer will be the plasma.
- The next thin layer is the buffy coat made of white blood cells and platelets.
- The bottom layer is red blood cells.

ALIQUOTING

Aliquoting a sample is done to withdraw serum or plasma from whole blood and/or to divide one sample into multiple aliquots for different tests. The individual must apply PPI, including gloves and goggles, and prepare aliquot tubes with appropriate labels. Aliquoting is done after centrifugation, with anticoagulated tubes aliquoted into plasma specimens and coagulated tubes aliquoted into serum specimens. It is necessary to place the centrifuged tubes into a rack and to avoid inverting the sample after centrifugation because this will cause remixing. A disposable pipette (never use a mouth pipette) is used to transfer each aliquot, starting from the top of the sample and working downward toward the point of separation. The aliquots are transferred to labeled tubes. As soon as an aliquot tube is filled, it must be capped. Aliquoted samples must be carefully labeled because serum and plasma are indistinguishable once they are aliquoted. Some other types of samples, such as saliva, must be mixed using a vortex mixer prior to aliquoting to ensure the sample is homogenous. Aliquots should be placed promptly in the appropriate storage, such as the refrigerator or -20 °C or -80 °C freezer.

TEMPERATURE REQUIREMENTS FOR SPECIMENS

Specimen storage is often at room temperature, which is generally based on the range found in temperature-controlled buildings: 20-25 °C. Blood bank and laboratory specimen refrigerators are maintained at 2-4 °C. Freezers are maintained at -20 °C with some specialty freezers at -80 °C. Incubators provide for a range of temperatures with much incubation done at 37 °C (body temperature). Samples may remain viable for different periods of time, depending on how they are stored. Some serum and plasma samples must be frozen prior to shipping. Temperature requirements depend on the type of specimen and the test.

Transport with heat block at 37 °C: Cryoglobulins, cryofibrinogen, and cold agglutinin.

The most appropriate way to **chill a specimen** is to immerse it into an ice and water slush. Ice cubes alone will not allow for adequate cooling of the specimen, and the specimen may freeze where the ice cubes touch it, resulting in possible hemolysis or breakdown of the analyte. **Transport in ice slurry and refrigerate the following samples**: ACTH, acetone, ACE, ammonia, blood gases, catecholamines, FFA, gastrin, glucagon, homocysteine, lactic acid, PTH, blood pH, pyruvate, renin.

INVERTING A TUBE

A tube should be inverted if it contains an additive and if the manufacturer's instructions require it to be inverted. If the sample is in a nonadditive tube then it does not have to be inverted. An additive tube usually is inverted 3-8 times to properly mix the additive with the blood.

PREVENTING AEROSOL FORMATION WHEN STOPPER HAS NO SAFETY FEATURE TO PREVENT AEROSOL

The stopper should be covered with 4×4-inch gauze and placed behind a safety shield to ensure the aerosol is not inhaled. Proper protective clothing should be worn as well. A safety stopper removal device may also be used.

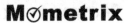

TIME CONSIDERATIONS WHEN PROCESSING SAMPLES

Specimens should be delivered to the laboratory for processing as quickly as possible and within no more than 45 minutes. Stat tests should be run first. Some tests have **time considerations** that must be followed:

- Blood gases must be processed within 20 minutes.
- Prothrombin time (PT) must be run on unrefrigerated blood sample within 24 hours.
- Partial thromboplastin time (PTT) must be run on a room temperature or refrigerated sample within 4 hours.

Additives also affect time considerations:

Additive	Tests	Time from collection
EDTA	Blood smear	Within 1 hour.
EDTA	CBC	Within 6 hours at room temperature and within 4 hours for micro-collection tubes. However, sample is usually stable at room temperature for 24 hours.
EDTA	ESR	Within 4 hours at room temperature and within 12 hours if refrigerated.
EDTA	Reticulocyte count	Within 6 hours at room temperature and within 72 hours if refrigerated.
Sodium fluoride	Glucose	Within 24 hours at room temperature and within 48 hours if refrigerated.

NHA Phlebotomy Practice Test #1

Want to take this practice test in an online interactive format?
Check out the bonus page, which includes interactive practice questions and
much more: **mometrix.com/bonus948/nhaphleb**

1. Following capillary blood collection, a bandage should be applied to the heel or finger of patients who are _____.

    a. 2 years or older
    b. 1 year or older
    c. 6 months or older
    d. 3 months or older

2. If a child weighs 34 lb, the maximum volume of blood that can be drawn in a 24-hr period is _____.

    a. 25 mL
    b. 50 mL
    c. 100 mL
    d. 200 mL

3. If a patient is undergoing analysis of gastric fluids before and after a gastric stimulant, for what blood test is the phlebotomist likely to need to collect a specimen?

    a. CBC.
    b. Uric acid.
    c. Serum gastrin.
    d. Albumin.

4. The most common reason for rejecting a specimen for chemistry is _____.

    a. an underfilled tube
    b. an overfilled tube
    c. clotting
    d. hemolysis

5. One of the reasons that serum is more often used for testing than plasma is that serum contains _____.

    a. more antigens
    b. fewer antigens
    c. more anticoagulants
    d. fewer gases

6. The primary function of leukocytes is to _____.

    a. oxygenate the cells
    b. carry solutes
    c. promote coagulation
    d. neutralize or destroy pathogens

7. If a patient complains of nausea after a blood draw, the most appropriate response is to _____.

    a. reassure the patient that the venipuncture is completed
    b. give the patient an emesis basin and encourage deep breathing
    c. give the patient a drink of cold water
    d. put the patient into the flat supine position

8. If a patient is heavily tattooed on both arms, from shoulders to wrists, with no areas left open, the most appropriate site for venipuncture is _____.

    a. any site
    b. the antecubital area with the oldest tattoos
    c. the dorsal metacarpal veins
    d. an area without solid dye

9. All lab samples should be handled according to _____.

    a. airborne precautions
    b. contact precautions
    c. universal precautions
    d. standard precautions

10. When a fasting urine test is ordered for glucose testing, this requires that which one of the following be collected?

    a. Any urine specimen after a specified period of fasting.
    b. The first urine specimen voided after a specified period of fasting.
    c. The second urine specimen voided after a specified period of fasting.
    d. The third urine specimen voided after a specified period of fasting.

11. When selecting an antecubital vein, priority should be given to veins in the _____.

    a. lateral aspect
    b. medial aspect
    c. median aspect
    d. lateral or medial aspect

12. Which of the following panels of tests may provide the best information about a patient with suspected liver dysfunction?

    a. BMP
    b. CMP
    c. Lipid profile
    d. Electrolyte panel

13. The best time to obtain a blood specimen for lowest cortisol level is at about_____.

    a. Noon
    b. Midnight
    c. 5 AM
    d. 8 PM

14. If a patient falls and experiences a fractured hip, the phlebotomist expects the patient will be treated in the _____.

    a. oncology department
    b. outpatient department
    c. orthopedic department
    d. obstetric department

15. Which of the following is NOT a cause of hemolysis?

    a. Failing to air dry antiseptic
    b. Using a larger-than-needed needle
    c. Using a smaller-than-needed needle
    d. Shaking tubes vigorously

16. During venipuncture, the correct position for the needle is _____.

    a. bevel up at a 30-degree angle to the skin
    b. bevel up at a 45-degree angle to the skin
    c. bevel down at a 30-degree angle to the skin
    d. bevel down at a 45-degree angle to the skin

17. The primary organization/agency that accredits laboratories and publishes laboratory checklists is _____.

    a. CLSI
    b. CAP
    c. FDA
    d. CDC

18. A used disposable needle and syringe should _____.

    a. have the needle bent to prevent further use
    b. have the needle recapped to prevent injury
    c. have the needle separated from the syringe
    d. be placed as is in a puncture-resistant sharps container

19. The main component of erythrocytes is _____.

    a. hemoglobin
    b. albumin
    c. sodium
    d. antibodies

20. Which of the following is NOT a good solution to the dealing with nonstandard shift work, such as 11 PM to 7 AM?

    a. Maintain different sleep patterns for working and nonworking days
    b. Schedule regular naptimes
    c. Avoid caffeinated beverages up to 6 hours before scheduled bedtime
    d. Use room-darkening shades while sleeping.

21. If a specimen must be chilled, the best method is to _____.
    a. place it in a water-and-ice mixture
    b. cover it with ice
    c. refrigerate it
    d. place it in dry ice

22. Serum differs from plasma in that serum _____.
    a. does not contain fibrinogen and clotting factors
    b. contains fibrinogen and clotting factors
    c. activates fibrinogen and clotting factors
    d. does not activate fibrinogen and clotting factors

23. Which one of the following situations introduces the most risk for error relating to patient ID?
    a. Older adult patient.
    b. Adolescent patient.
    c. Having multiple patients in one room.
    d. Outpatient.

24. Which one of the following POC tests measures the volume of RBCs in a patient's blood?
    a. Hgb.
    b. Hct.
    c. INR.
    d. Na.

25. The most commonly used needle gauge for venipuncture is _____.
    a. 19
    b. 21
    c. 23
    d. 24

26. A venipuncture should never be carried out proximal to a PICC line because _____.
    a. the blood will be diluted
    b. the catheter may be damaged
    c. doing so increases the risk of thrombophlebitis
    d. a large discard volume is required

27. When collecting a blood specimen from a patient in an isolation room, the phlebotomist should place the collection tray _____.
    a. at the nurse's station or another secured area
    b. on a table or chair outside of the room
    c. on a table or chair immediately inside the room
    d. on the bedside table

28. When collecting a blood specimen for trace elements, such as zinc, the appropriate tube type is _____.

    a. plastic
    b. element-free
    c. glass
    d. stopper-free

29. The primary focus of CLIA (1988) is to ensure that _____.

    a. patients get correct laboratory results
    b. patients are reimbursed for errors
    c. patients are informed of rights
    d. patients are protected from injury

30. The volume of blood that a Microtainer® holds is _____.

    a. 0.25 mL
    b. 0.5 mL
    c. 0.75 mL
    d. 1 mL

31. When carrying out a rapid test for group A *Streptococci* from a throat swab, if there is no blue control line on the dipstick at 5 minutes, this means that _____.

    a. the test is positive
    b. the test is negative
    c. the test is inconclusive
    d. the test is invalid

32. Which one of the following is an appropriate question to verify a patient's ID?

    a. "Is your name Sally Evans?"
    b. "Are you Ms. Evans? What is your birthdate?"
    c. "Ms. Evans, were you born on March 16, 1980?"
    d. "Can you tell me your name and birthdate?"

33. A patient with an order for blood tests has a clamped PICC line in the left arm, so the phlebotomist should draw blood from the _____.

    a. Right arm
    b. Left arm, distal to the PICC line
    c. Left arm, proximal to the PICC line
    d. PICC line

34. During a blood draw and collection in multiple vacuum tubes, if the third tube fails to fill, the most appropriate initial response is to _____.

    a. insert the needle deeper into the vein
    b. discontinue the venipuncture and try a different site
    c. try a different vacuum tube
    d. call for assistance

35. Blood specimens for ammonia levels should be separated from the cells and tested within _____.

    a. 15 minutes
    b. 30 minutes
    c. 60 minutes
    d. 4 hours

36. The infections most commonly transmitted through needlestick and sharp injuries are _____.

    a. HBV, HCV, and HIV
    b. HBV, HIV, and HZV
    c. HIV, syphilis, and CMV
    d. HBV, HB, and HZV

37. The most common plasma protein is _____.

    a. fibrinogen
    b. albumin
    c. alpha globulin
    d. beta globulin

38. If a phlebotomist accidentally experiences a slight needlestick that does not draw blood after obtaining a blood sample, the phlebotomist should _____.

    a. wash the site with soap and water and take no further action
    b. wipe the site with an alcohol swab and verify that there is no bleeding
    c. wash the site with soap and water and report the incident
    d. flush the site with running water for 20 minutes and report the incident

39. If a biohazard sign at the entrance to the laboratory lists the laboratory's biosafety level as 3 (BSL-3), this means that the lab studies infectious agents that _____.

    a. do not consistently cause human disease
    b. pose a risk if inhaled, swallowed, or exposed to the skin
    c. are airborne and could potentially cause lethal disease
    d. are airborne, lethal, and for which there is no effective treatment

40. The purpose of a blood transfer device is to prevent _____.

    a. specimen contamination
    b. a needlestick
    c. tube breakage
    d. spillage

41. If a patient in the emergency department refuses to have blood drawn but the phlebotomist does so at the physician's assistance, the phlebotomist may be charged with _____.

    a. assault
    b. negligence
    c. malpractice
    d. nothing

42. Which of the following hazardous label colors is used to indicate a substance that is reactive, normally stable but may become unstable and dangerous if heated?

   a. Blue
   b. White
   c. Yellow
   d. Red

43. If a patient has undergone bilateral mastectomies with surgeries 5 years apart, what venipuncture site should the phlebotomist select?

   a. An ankle on either side.
   b. The phlebotomist should ask the physician for instructions.
   c. The arm on the side of the most recent mastectomy.
   d. The arm on the side of the most distant mastectomy.

44. Which of the following factors is likely to have the greatest effect on the results of a CBC processed within 2 hours of collection of the sample?

   a. Mealtime
   b. Mild exercise
   c. Environmental temperature
   d. Dehydration

45. When collecting a blood specimen from an ambulatory patient in the home environment, the patient should be placed _____.

   a. in a comfortable chair
   b. sitting at a table
   c. recumbent or in a chair with arm supports
   d. lying supine in bed

46. If a venipuncture is done on the basilic vein and the blood returns bright red and appears to pulse, this indicates _____.

   a. Accidental arterial draw
   b. High blood pressure
   c. Blood abnormality
   d. Successful blood draw

47. How long should the phlebotomist observe a venipuncture site for signs of excessive or persistent bleeding before applying a bandage?

   a. 1–2 seconds.
   b. 3–5 seconds.
   c. 5–10 seconds.
   d. 10–20 seconds.

48. If a patient has severely impaired circulation in the legs and has had a recent bilateral mastectomy, the best choice for a blood draw is probably _____.

   a. Foot or ankle veins
   b. Artery
   c. Dominant arm
   d. Nondominant arm

49. Which of the following blood cells does NOT contain a nucleus?

    a. Neutrophil
    b. Lymphocyte
    c. Erythrocyte
    d. Platelet

50. Which one of the following tests requires a timed specimen?

    a. CBC.
    b. Uric acid.
    c. Blood culture.
    d. Cortisol.

51. Which of the following is NOT a characteristic of a safety feature for a venipuncture needle?

    a. Activation is from behind needle
    b. Activation requires one hand only
    c. May be detachable
    d. Provides permanent containment

52. If a patient had a right mastectomy 6 months ago, blood may be drawn from the _____.

    a. left arm
    b. left or right ankle
    c. right arm—distal area only
    d. left or right arm

53. When performing a venipuncture on a patient under investigation (PUI) for Ebola, the correct isolation procedure is _____.

    a. contact
    b. droplet
    c. contact and droplet
    d. standard, contact, and droplet plus enhanced measures

54. At room temperature, complete clotting usually occurs within _____.

    a. 10–15 minutes
    b. 15–30 minutes
    c. 30–60 minutes
    d. 60–90 minutes

55. RBCs normally circulate in the bloodstream for _____.

    a. 60 days
    b. 90 days
    c. 120 days
    d. 150 days

56. During a venipuncture, if the patient cries out and complains of severe pain, the most appropriate response is to _____.

    a. quickly finish the draw
    b. ask the patient to rate the pain on a scale of 1-10
    c. encourage the patient to take a deep breath and relax
    d. immediately remove the needle

57. A micro-sample is generally collected from a 9-month-old infant by _____.

    a. finger stick
    b. scalp stick
    c. heel stick
    d. venipuncture

58. If a patient jerks the arm as the venipuncture needle is removed, resulting in a needlestick of the patient with only a very small drop of blood, the most important action is to _____.

    a. Bandage the needlestick
    b. Follow needlestick protocol
    c. Do nothing more
    d. Notify the patient's nurse

59. If a patient with rheumatoid arthritis has severe flexion contractures of both arms and hands, the best solution for selecting a venipuncture site is probably to _____.

    a. Ask the patient
    b. Use the nondominant hand
    c. Use the foot or ankle
    d. Suggest an arterial draw

60. If a sample is designated QNS, this means that _____.

    a. the quality is not standardized
    b. the quality is nonsterile
    c. the quantity is not standardized
    d. the quantity is not sufficient

61. After collecting a blood sample, a tube containing sodium citrate as an additive should be inverted _____.

    a. 1–3 times
    b. 3–4 times
    c. 4–6 times
    d. 5–10 times

62. At which of the following times are peak levels of cortisol usually obtained?

    a. In the late afternoon
    b. Around noon
    c. In the early morning
    d. At midnight

63. If a patient sitting in a chair has a generalized convulsive seizure during venipuncture, the appropriate response is to discontinue venipuncture and _____.

    a. call for help to ease the patient to the floor
    b. restrain the patient in the chair
    c. support the patient in the chair and call 9-1-1
    d. place a tongue blade between the patient's teeth

64. If, after filling a collection tube, the phlebotomist notes blood on the outside of a collection tube, the correct action is to _____.

    a. Discard the specimen in a biohazard waste container
    b. Wipe tube with disinfectant and seal in a biohazard bag
    c. Discard the specimen in a sharps container
    d. Transport to lab in gloved hand

65. When collecting a specimen from a patient in a long-term-care facility, the first thing the phlebotomist should do is to _____.

    a. knock on the patient's door
    b. check in at the nursing station
    c. contact the patient prior to arrival
    d. enter the patient's room

66. When using a portable heat block to maintain a blood specimen at body temperature, the phlebotomist should expect the heat block to hold the temperature for approximately _____.

    a. 5 minutes
    b. 15 minutes
    c. 60 minutes
    d. 2 hours

67. Control runs of automated systems should be carried out _____.

    a. monthly
    b. weekly
    c. at the end of each day
    d. at the beginning of each day

68. Serum specimens can be centrifuged _____.

    a. before clotting occurs
    b. after clotting is completed
    c. at any stage of clotting
    d. immediately upon receipt

69. Phlebotomists are especially at risk for developing an allergic response to _____.

    a. latex
    b. alcohol
    c. plastic
    d. nitrile

70. For most POC pregnancy tests, the earliest time to take the test for accuracy is _____.

a. any time
b. 14 days after unprotected sex
c. 1 week after a missed period
d. 1 day after a missed period

71. The total blood volume of a child is approximately _____.

a. 65–70 mL/kg
b. 75–80 mL/kg
c. 85–105 mL/kg
d. 100–120 mL/kg

72. With RIDTs, positive or negative test results are more likely to be accurate if the sample is obtained within _____.

a. 1 day of the onset of symptoms
b. 2 days of the onset of symptoms
c. 4 days of the onset of symptoms
d. 7 days of the onset of symptoms

73. When decanting a 24-hour urine specimen, which may splash, into a sink to a sanitary sewer, the phlebotomist should _____.

a. run water while decanting
b. pour from a height of at least 6 inches
c. stand as far away from the sink as possible
d. wear facial protection and a fluid-proof apron

74. Which antiseptic is most commonly used for cleaning the venipuncture site?

a. Chlorhexidine gluconate.
b. Povidone-iodine.
c. Isopropyl alcohol 70%.
d. Isopropyl alcohol 90%.

75. The maximum number of samples or tests that can be performed each hour by an assay system is the _____.

a. input
b. throughput
c. output
d. continuous flow

76. The additive that is most effective at preserving coagulation factors is _____.

a. Potassium oxalate
b. Lithium heparin
c. Na_2EDTA
d. Sodium citrate

77. For therapeutic drug monitoring, the peak time for most drugs after intramuscular injection is approximately _____.

   a. 30 minutes
   b. 60 minutes
   c. 90 minutes
   d. 2 hours

78. If a patient reports a history of episodes of syncope, the most appropriate response is to _____.

   a. place the patient in a recumbent position
   b. encourage the patient to do deep breathing and relaxation exercises
   c. reassure the patient that venipuncture is not painful
   d. provide smelling salts (ammonia inhalant)

79. Strenuous exercise may increase values of which of the following tests for more than 24 hours?

   a. Aldosterone
   b. Lactic acid
   c. Albumin
   d. Lactic dehydrogenase (LD)

80. If peritoneal fluid is aspirated during a paracentesis and must be tested for cell counts, which type of specimen tube is indicated?

   a. EDTA.
   b. Sodium fluoride.
   c. Heparin.
   d. Nonanticoagulant.

81. If the phlebotomist tells a friend about doing a venipuncture for a famous actor who is hospitalized, this constitutes _____.

   a. a HIPAA violation
   b. malpractice
   c. slander
   d. battery

82. If a patient must do a 72-hour stool collection for fecal fat analysis, the stool should be kept under what conditions during the collection period?

   a. At room temperature.
   b. Under refrigeration.
   c. Frozen in separate bags for each day.
   d. In a heated container.

83. If CSF is collected in four numbered containers, the first tube is used for _____.

   a. microbiology studies
   b. cell count and differential
   c. cytology and special tests
   d. chemistry and immunology tests

84. **If a person's blood is type O, what plasma agglutinin is present in the person's blood?**
    a. Anti-A.
    b. Anti-B.
    c. Anti-A and anti-B.
    d. None.

85. **When venipuncture is done in edematous tissue, the results will likely be _____.**
    a. the same as those from normal tissue
    b. inconclusive
    c. contaminated with bacteria
    d. altered

86. **Black-capped collection tubes are used only for _____.**
    a. toxicology
    b. lead levels
    c. coagulation tests
    d. ESR

87. **If category B infectious materials must be transported out of the area for testing, specimens must not exceed _____.**
    a. 200 mL or 200 g
    b. 300 mL or 300 g
    c. 400 mL or 400 g
    d. 500 mL or 500 g

88. **Which pattern of antecubital veins is predominant in most populations?**
    a. The M pattern.
    b. The N pattern.
    c. The H pattern.
    d. An atypical pattern.

89. **When conducting the urine dipstick test, how should the dipstick be held after dipping it into the urine sample and withdrawing it?**
    a. Maintained in the urine.
    b. Vertically so the urine drips quickly.
    c. Horizontally so the urine pools.
    d. Diagonally so the urine drips slowly.

90. **When obtaining a blood specimen for coagulation tests (PT, aPTT), when is the use of a discard tube indicated?**
    a. It is never indicated when obtaining a blood specimen for coagulation tests.
    b. It is always indicated when obtaining a blood specimen for coagulation tests.
    c. It is indicated whenever the coagulation tube is the first tube needed.
    d. It is indicated when a winged (butterfly) blood collection set is used and the coagulation tube is filled first.

91. Which one of the following actions may result in hemolysis of a specimen?

    a. Collecting a specimen from a VAD.
    b. Using a 22-gauge needle for collection.
    c. Leaving the tourniquet in place for 45 seconds.
    d. Gently inverting the specimen.

92. If a blood specimen is to be obtained for the trough level of a drug, the best time to draw the blood is usually _____.

    a. 15 minutes before the next scheduled dose
    b. 30 minutes before the next scheduled dose
    c. 60 minutes before the next scheduled dose
    d. 2 hours after the last scheduled dose

93. When doing a venipuncture, the correct angle of insertion of the needle is usually _____.

    a. 10 degrees
    b. 20 degrees
    c. 30 degrees
    d. 45 degrees

94. If blood is withdrawn for noncoagulation studies from a VAD, this requires _____.

    a. waiting at least 60 minutes after a heparin flush before withdrawing blood
    b. drawing a discard tube before withdrawing blood
    c. flushing the VAD with preservative-free NS and drawing a discard tube first
    d. flushing the VAD with preservative-free NS before withdrawing blood

95. The most abundant electrolytes in plasma are sodium and _____.

    a. chloride
    b. potassium
    c. calcium
    d. magnesium

96. Lymph fluid is similar in compensation to _____.

    a. Bile
    b. Plasma
    c. Chyme
    d. Serum

97. Tests that are not appropriate for delivery to the lab by pneumatic tube include _____.

    a. albumin
    b. glucose
    c. cryoglobulins
    d. uric acid

98. If a phlebotomist develops dermatitis from all types of gloves, the best solution is to _____.

    a. Stop wearing gloves
    b. Double wash the hands only
    c. Use glove liners or barrier cream
    d. Wear gloves as briefly as possible

99. If the safety device on the venipuncture needle fails to activate, leaving the needle exposed, in order to dispose of the needle, the phlebotomist should _____.

    a. place the cap back on the needle
    b. bend and break the needle
    c. wrap a gauze pad around the needle
    d. carefully place the needle in the sharps container

100. If less than the recommended volume necessary for blood cultures is obtained, how should the blood be distributed in the aerobic and anaerobic specimen tubes?

    a. Place equal amounts in the aerobic and anaerobic specimen tubes.
    b. Fill only the aerobic specimen tube.
    c. Fill the aerobic specimen tube completely, and place the remainder in the anaerobic tube.
    d. Fill the anaerobic specimen tube completely, and place the remainder in the aerobic tube.

101. All laboratory testing in the United States, except for research testing, is regulated by the Centers for Medicare and Medicaid Services through the _____.

    a. AHA
    b. CLIA
    c. CDC
    d. OIG

102. The maximum volume of blood that may be drawn from a 20 lb infant in an eight-week period is _____.

    a. 20 mL
    b. 60 mL
    c. 100 mL
    d. 140 mL

103. Which one of the following tests requires that the specimen be chilled?

    a. Potassium
    b. CBC
    c. Uric acid
    d. Lactic acid

104. "DNR" means _____.

    a. Do not record
    b. Does not remember
    c. Does not respond
    d. Do not resuscitate

105. At room temperature, EDTA specimens for ESR should be tested within _____.

a. 1 hour
b. 2 hours
c. 4 hours
d. 6 hours

106. Mouth pipetting of a blood sample is _____,

a. Used for skin punctures only
b. Optional
c. Reserved for pathologists only
d. Prohibited

107. The POC test that is most accurate for monitoring heparin therapy is _____.

a. PT
b. ACT
c. INR
d. aPTT

108. Warning signs, such as "fall precautions," are usually placed on the_____.

a. Foot of the patient's bed
b. Wall behind the patient's head
c. Patient's door
d. Patient's armband

109. The nerve most often injured with venipuncture is the _____.

a. radial
b. ulnar
c. musculocutaneous
d. median

110. When collecting a capillary blood sample after a fingerstick or heelstick, it is generally necessary to _____.

a. wipe away the first drop
b. collect every drop
c. "milk" the finger or heel to promote blood flow
d. scrape the collector against the skin to collect the dripping blood

111. If the needle hits the median nerve during an antecubital venipuncture, the most common patient complaint is _____.

a. Numbness
b. Dull aching pain
c. Muscle twitching
d. Severe shock-like pain

112. Which one of the following types of POC tests is used to determine a patient's response to aspirin therapy?

    a. PT/INR.
    b. ACT.
    c. aPTT.
    d. Platelet function.

113. Gloves should generally be donned prior to _____.

    a. placing the tourniquet
    b. cleansing the skin
    c. palpating the veins
    d. performing the venipuncture

114. A blood specimen for a CBC should be collected in a tube that contains _____.

    a. No additive
    b. ACD
    c. Na_2EDTA
    d. Clot activator

115. Hemostasis refers to _____.

    a. stoppage of bleeding
    b. clotting of blood
    c. loss of blood
    d. concentration of blood

116. If, after leaving a patient's room, the phlebotomist is asked by the patient's brother what tests the patient is having, the phlebotomist should _____.

    a. provide information
    b. provide no information
    c. deny having any knowledge
    d. ask the patient's permission to divulge

117. When the phlebotomist enters an isolation room to draw blood, the phlebotomy tray should be_____.

    a. covered with a sterile drape
    b. placed on a table inside the room
    c. left outside the room
    d. replaced after leaving the room

118. Which one of the following test specimens is photosensitive and must be protected from exposure to light?

    a. Cryobilinogen.
    b. Bilirubin.
    c. Pyruvate.
    d. ACTH.

119. If a patient has made a fist for venipuncture, at what point should he or she generally be instructed to open the hand?

    a. after the needle is inserted.
    b. when blood flow is established.
    c. after the collection is completed.
    d. after the needle is removed.

120. When having trouble visualizing a vein, the best approach is to _____.

    a. ask the patient to pump the fist
    b. vigorously massage the area of the vein
    c. leave the tourniquet in place for 2 minutes
    d. ask the patient to make a fist

Answer Key and Explanations for Test #1

1. A: Following capillary blood collection, a bandage should be applied to the heel or finger of patients who are 2 years old or older. Newborns and infants younger than 2 should not be bandaged because the bandage may pose a choking risk because of the child's tendency to put things in the mouth, and the skin is too friable and may become irritated or tear when the bandage is removed.

2. B: CLSI guidelines recommend for pediatric patients that the amount of blood drawn in 24 hours be no more than 5% of the patient's total blood volume, using 65-70 mL/kg as the estimate for blood volume.

$$34 \text{ lb} \times \frac{1 \text{ kg}}{2.2 \text{ lb}} = 15.45 \text{ kg}$$

$$15.45 \text{ kg} \times 65 \frac{\text{mL}}{\text{kg}} = 1005 \text{ mL}$$

5% of that total volume would be approximately 50 mL, the maximum volume of blood that can be drawn in 24 hours for this patient. Care must be taken to avoid withdrawing more than 5% of the child's total blood volume in a 24-hr period. Additionally, the phlebotomist must consider the maximum amount of blood volume that can be withdrawn within other time periods. CLSI regulations limit the amount of blood drawn over an 8-week period to no more than 10% of the patient's total blood volume.

3. C: If a patient is undergoing analysis of gastric fluids before and after a gastric stimulant, the blood test that the phlebotomist is likely to need to collect a specimen for is serum gastrin, which evaluates gastric production. The serum is collected in a red- or gray-topped tube. Gastric fluid analysis and serum gastrin are tested to help diagnose chronic gastritis, chronic renal failure, gastric and duodenal ulcers, gastric carcinoma, G-cell hyperplasia, pernicious anemia, pyloric obstruction, and hyperparathyroidism.

4. D: The most common reason for rejecting a specimen for chemistry is hemolysis, whereas the most common reason for hematology is clotting. Other reasons that specimens may be rejected include overfilling or underfilling a tube because this alters the required ratio of additive to specimen and can interfere with the testing results. Specimens transported and handled in the wrong collection tube, at the wrong temperature, with the wrong additive, or with exposure to light (if photosensitive) may also be rejected.

5. A: One of the reasons that serum is more often used for testing than plasma is that serum contains more antigens, so it can be used to carry out a wider variety of tests. Additionally, anticoagulants found in plasma may interfere with some tests. While plasma may be administered as transfusions, serum is much more commonly used for testing, although in some cases, a test can be done with either plasma or serum.

6. D: The primary function of leukocytes (white blood cells) is to neutralize or destroy pathogens through phagocytosis (engulfing and destroying) or the production of antibodies. There are five types of leukocytes:

Neutrophils	54–62%	Destroy pathogens with phagocytosis.
Eosinophils	≤3%	Ingest/Detoxify foreign protein.
Basophils	<1%	Release histamine and heparin, and promote an inflammatory response.
Lymphocytes	24–38%	T-cells attack infected cells; B-cells produce antibodies.
Monocytes	3–7%	Destroy pathogens with phagocytosis.

7. B: If a patient complains of nausea after a blood draw, the most appropriate response is to give the patient an emesis basin (because nausea often leads to vomiting) and encourage deep breathing because this sometimes eases nausea. A cool, damp cloth may also be applied to the patient's forehead. In most cases, nausea subsides within a few moments, but first-aid personnel should be notified. If the patient is lying flat and supine, he or she should be turned to one side to avoid aspiration if vomiting occurs.

8. C: If a patient is heavily tattooed on both arms, from shoulders to wrists with no areas left open, the most appropriate site for venipuncture is the dorsal metacarpal veins. Tattooed areas should be avoided if possible because they may harbor infection (if done recently) and may mask signs of inflammation or bruising. If it is necessary to withdraw blood from a tattooed area, it is important to try to find an area that is open and free of dye, especially solid-dyed areas.

9. D: All lab samples should be handled according to standard precautions, which combine universal precautions and body substance precautions because of the concern that not all infectious processes are obvious or identified. With body substance isolation, gloves must be worn for all contact with blood, body fluids, and any moist body surface such as mucous membranes. With universal precautions, all blood and body fluids are considered potentially infectious. Standard precautions also require respiratory hygiene/cough etiquette.

10. C: When a fasting urine test is ordered for glucose testing, this means that the second urine specimen voided after a specified period of fasting should be collected, usually 8 hours. The first specimen, which is affected by food eaten before the fasting period, is discarded. If a first-voiding specimen is ordered, it is usually collected first thing in the morning after approximately 8 hours of sleep. First-voiding specimens are usually more concentrated than subsequent voids. Random urine specimens may be obtained at any time.

11. C: When selecting an antecubital vein, priority should be given to veins in the median (middle) aspect. These include the median vein and the lateral aspect of the median cubital vein. If these are not satisfactory, the next to consider are the veins in the lateral (outer) aspect, including the cephalic vein and the accessory cephalic vein, although there is increased risk of injury to the lateral nerve. The last to consider are the veins in the medial (inner) aspect. These include the basilic vein and the medial aspect of the median cubital vein. Venipuncture in these veins poses increased risk of injury to the brachial artery and median antebrachial cutaneous nerves.

12. B: The CMP (comprehensive metabolic panel) contains the tests found in the BMP (basic metabolic panel) (blood urea nitrogen [BUN], Ca, CO_2, Cl, creatinine, glucose, K, and Na) as well additional tests that give information about liver function (albumin, ALP, AST, bilirubin, and total protein). While these are fewer specific tests than found in the liver function panel, the CMP is often used to screen for live dysfunction and, if tests are positive, then further testing may be ordered.

13. B: The best time to obtain a blood specimen for lowest cortisol level is at about midnight. Increased levels of cortisol indicate adrenal hyperfunction and Cushing syndrome while decreased levels indicate hypofunction and Addison's disease. Cortisol levels exhibit diurnal variation, usually peaking in the early morning (about 8 AM) and reaching the lowest level around midnight, so multiple tests may be ordered at different times. If cortisol tests are abnormal, then additional tests are usually ordered to confirm a diagnosis.

14. C: If a patient falls and experiences a fractured hip, the phlebotomist expects the patient will be treated in the orthopedic department, which specializes in caring for patients with impairments of or injuries to the skeletal system, including fractures. The oncology department specializes in the care of patients with cancer. Obstetrics specializes in the care of pregnant women, including labor and delivery. Outpatient departments, also commonly known as ambulatory care centers, provide same-day treatment and surgical procedures without hospital inpatient admission.

15. B: Using a larger-than-needed needle does not result in hemolysis (rupturing of RBCs), but using too small of a needle may. Other causes of hemolysis include failing to air dry the antiseptic before venipuncture, withdrawing blood from the area of a hematoma, shaking the collection tube instead of inverting to mix the blood with additive, rapidly emptying blood from a syringe into a collection tube, and withdrawing the plunger on a syringe too forcefully.

16. A: During venipuncture, the correct position for the needle is bevel up at a 30-degree angle to the skin. Inserting at too steep of an angle can result in the needle being inserted too far, and this increases the risk of damage to nerves and arteries. However, if the needle is not inserted deeply enough, it may miss the vein. This may occur in patients whose veins are especially deep or in patients who are markedly obese.

17. B: The primary organization/agency that accredits laboratories and publishes laboratory checklists is the College of American Pathologists (CAP). CAP accreditation is voluntary, but to qualify, labs must meet standards established in the checklists. CAP produces checklists utilizing standards produced by the Clinical Laboratory Standards Institute (CLSI). Laboratories that are CAP accredited are usually exempt from inspection by government agencies because they are considered in compliance with requirements established by the Clinical Laboratory Improvement Act.

18. D: A used disposable needle and syringe should be placed as is in a puncture-resistant sharps container. Needles should not be bent, recapped, or separated from the syringe because any handling of the needle introduces the risk of a needlestick injury. Needles and syringes should be placed in the sharps container immediately after use whenever possible. Sharps that are nondisposable must be placed in a hard-walled container and taken to the processing area to be decontaminated.

19. A: The main component of erythrocytes (RBCs) is hemoglobin. Hemoglobin is a complex protein that contains iron; it carries oxygen throughout the body and carries CO_2 back to the lungs. Erythrocytes are the most plentiful blood cells with 4.5–5 million per cubic milliliter of blood. They are concave discs that lack nuclei and have a life expectancy of approximately 120 days. Erythrocytes are produced in the bone marrow in a process called erythropoiesis.

20. A: Because it is difficult for the body to adjust to different sleep times, the person working a nontraditional shift, such as 11 PM to 7 AM, should try to maintain the same sleep patterns for both working and nonworking days. Additionally, scheduling a short daily nap and avoiding caffeinated beverages up to 6 hours before scheduled bedtime may help the person get adequate sleep. Keeping the bedroom dark, such as with room-darkening shades, during sleeping hours may help the person get adequate sleep.

21. A: If a specimen must be chilled, the best method is to place the specimen in a water-and-ice mixture so that adequate contact is made. Placing it in or on ice alone is not adequate because the cold will not be applied uniformly. Refrigerating the item cools it too slowly, and placing it in dry ice poses the risk that hemolysis may occur because of the extreme temperature change. Whole blood specimens are not usually chilled.

22. A: Serum differs from plasma in that serum does not contain fibrinogen and other clotting factors. Serum is the extracellular liquid portion of plasma, minus fibrinogen, clotting factors, and blood cells. However, serum does contain solutes (proteins, minerals, hormones, gases) and is important as a source of electrolytes. Serum is the product of centrifugation of coagulated blood and consists of 90% water. Serum is commonly used for chemistry testing except for potassium because potassium is released into the serum during the clotting process, resulting in a higher level than in plasma.

23. C: Having multiple patients in one room introduces the most risk for error relating to patient ID because the order may include the wrong bed assignment, so it is especially important to double-check the patient's ID. Because patients may be confused, the wristband should always be checked to verify the person's name. Other situations that increase the risk of error include tests on siblings or twins, newborns, common names (Mary Jones), and names that look alike or sound alike.

24. B: Hct (hematocrit) (aka packed cell volume [PCV]) measures the volume of RBCs in a patient's blood. A small sample of anticoagulated blood is centrifuged; the results reflect the percentage of cells to liquid. The normal hematocrit value varies according to gender and age:

Age	Male	Female
0 to 1 week	46–68	46–68
1 to 2 months	32–54	32–54
3 months to 5 years	31–43	31–43
6 to 8 years	33–41	33–41
15 to adult	38–51	33–45
Older adult	36–52	34–46

25. B: The most commonly used needle gauge for venipuncture is 21. The size of the needle decreases with increasing numbers, so gauge 21 is larger than gauge 23. Using a needle larger than 21-gauge should be avoided because it may result in extra pain and has few benefits. If veins are smaller, then size 23 may be used, but smaller gauges may increase the risk of hemolysis and also increase the time needed to collect a specimen.

26. B: A venipuncture should never be carried out proximal to a peripherally inserted central catheter (PICC) line because the catheter may be damaged when the tourniquet is applied or the needle is inserted and could even break, causing fragments to migrate. If possible, the arm with a PICC line should be avoided for blood draws; however, if it is absolutely necessary, the tourniquet must be placed and the venipuncture is done distal to the PICC line.

27. A: When collecting a blood specimen from a patient in an isolation room, the phlebotomist should collect the needed supplies and place the collection tray at the nurse's station or in another secured area. The tray should not be left unattended in a public area. Any supplies taken into the isolation room are considered contaminated and cannot then be used for other patients, so they must be properly disposed of. Tourniquets used for isolation rooms should be dedicated to the patient or should be disposable.

28. B: When collecting a blood specimen for trace elements, such as zinc, selenium, or mercury, the appropriate tube type is element-free. These are specialty tubes designed so that they do not contaminate the sample with trace elements that are typically found in glass and plastic containers. These tubes usually have royal-blue tops and are available with EDTA or heparin, or they are free of additives. Samples for lead testing are collected in tan-topped tubes containing K2 EDTA.

29. A: The primary focus of CLIA (Clinical Laboratory Improvement Amendments) (1988) is to ensure that patients get correct laboratory results through requiring that laboratories meet quality standards. Laboratories are required to be certified by state authorities and by CMS (Center for Medicare and Medicaid Services). The three agencies that are responsible for CLIA are:

- FDA (Food and Drug Administration): Categorizes tests and develops rules.
- CMS: Issues certificates, inspects, publishes rules, and monitors lab performance.
- CDC (Centers for Disease Control and Prevention): Provides research, develops information, and manages the advisory committee (CLIAC).

30. B: Because Microtainer® tubes are used to collect very small volumes of capillary blood, such as from a fingerstick, they typically hold up to 0.5 mL of blood. These small containers, also sometimes referred to as "bullets" because of their miniature size, contain the same types of additives as larger evacuated tubes and the caps are color-coded in the same manner so that the additives can be easily identified.

31. D: When carrying out a rapid test for group A *Streptococci* from a throat swab, if there is no blue control line on the dipstick at 5 minutes, this means that the test is invalid, possibly because the dipstick if outdated. For the test, a tube is filled with three drops each of reagent A and B and the swab is placed into the tube for 1 minute and rotated at least five times before removal. The dipstick is then placed in the tube for 5 minutes. The blue control line must appear by 5 minutes for a valid test. A positive finding is a pink or purple test line.

32. D: An appropriate question to verify a patient's ID is "Can you tell me your name and birthdate?" Asking for direct information is important because if a patient is confused or hard of hearing, he or she may answer "yes" or "no" to questions incorrectly. For inpatients, the ID band should always be checked to verify the information that they provide. If patients do not have an ID band, common in the outpatient setting, then they should be asked to provide and spell their names and provide their birthdates.

33. A: A patient with an order for blood tests has a clamped peripherally inserted central catheter (PICC) line in the left arm, so the phlebotomist should draw blood from the right arm. Drawing blood from a vascular access device, such as a PICC line, is outside of the scope of practice of the phlebotomist; however, the phlebotomist may provide necessary collection tubes to a nurse or physician who accesses the PICC line and may transport the tubes. If a PICC line is in one arm, the alternate arm should be used for venipuncture if possible.

34. C: During a blood draw and collection in multiple vacuum tubes, if the third tube fails to fill, the most appropriate initial response is to try a different vacuum tube. Tubes sometimes lose their vacuum. If the new tube also does not fill, then the phlebotomist should check to make sure that the entire bevel of the needle is completely under the skin. If a new tube does not solve the problem and the needle is in the correct place, the venipuncture may need to be discontinued and a new site is tried.

35. A: Blood specimens for ammonia levels should be separated from the cells and tested within 15 minutes because the levels increase rapidly at room temperature. Specimens should be transported in an ice slurry or cooling tray and processed immediately. Blood ammonia levels are often checked to diagnose or monitor hepatic encephalopathy, which can result in toxic levels of ammonia. Other causes of increased ammonia include upper gastrointestinal tract bleeding, salicylate poisoning, liver failure, kidney disease, and parenteral nutrition.

36. A: The infections most commonly transmitted through needlestick and sharp injuries are HBV (hepatitis B virus), HCV (hepatitis C virus), and HIV (human immunodeficiency virus). While these viruses pose the greatest risk—and people may be co-infected, putting the person who has a needlestick or sharp injury at risk of more than one disease—other infectious disorders (more than 20) can also be spread through needlestick and sharp injury, including syphilis, HZV (herpes zoster virus), toxoplasmosis, TB, Rocky Mountain spotted fever, blastomycosis, and cutaneous gonorrhea.

37. B: The most common plasma protein is albumin. Plasma proteins help to regulate the movement of water between cells and blood, controlling blood volume and affecting blood pressure. Plasma proteins include:

- Albumin (60%): Produced in the liver and maintains colloid osmotic pressure.
- Globulins (36%): Alpha and beta globulins are both produced in the liver. They transport lipids and fat-soluble vitamins. Gamma globulins are produced in lymphatic tissue and act as immune antibodies.
- Fibrinogen (4%): Produced in the liver and involved in coagulation.

38. C: If a phlebotomist accidentally experiences a slight needlestick that does not draw blood after obtaining a blood sample, the phlebotomist should wash the site with soap and water. The incident must be reported as soon as possible to a supervisor, and needlestick protocol should be followed. This may include testing and/or prophylaxis, depending on the patient's health history. In some cases, the patient may also be tested for communicable diseases, such as HIV, in order to determine the risk to the phlebotomist.

39. C: If a biohazard sign at the entrance to the laboratory lists the laboratory's biosafety level as 3 (BSL-3), this means that the lab handles infectious agents that are airborne and could potentially cause lethal disease, such as COVID-19 and *Mycobacterium tuberculosis*. Biosafety levels:

- BSL-1: Infectious agents do not consistently cause disease.
- BSL-2: Infectious agents pose a risk if inhaled, swallowed, or exposed to the skin.
- BSL-3: As above.
- BSL-4: Infectious agents are airborne, lethal, and no effective treatment is available.

40. B: The purpose of a blood transfer device is to prevent a needlestick. The blood transfer device was devised when OSHA required that safety needles be used when collecting blood specimens. These needles cannot be used to inject blood into a collection tube, so the safety needle is removed and the transfer device, which contains a small needle inside, is attached to the Luer. The collection tube is then inserted into the transfer device and the blood is transferred when the needle penetrates the cap.

41. A: If a patient in the emergency department refuses to have blood drawn but the phlebotomist does so at the physician's assistance, the phlebotomist may be charged with assault. Unless a patient is a minor, legally deemed incompetent to make decisions, or is legally required to have a test (such as a blood alcohol level or tox-screen for illicit drugs), then the individual has an absolute right to refuse any and all treatments and procedures.

42. C: Most hazardous material comes with warning labels that are color-coded to indicate the type of risk, with NFPA (National Fire Protection Association) ratings ranging from 0 (no risk) to 4 (extreme risk):

- Yellow: reactive, normally stable (0) but becomes unstable if heated (1), may undergo a violent chemical reaction (2), post a severe risk of explosion (3), and extreme hazard if fire occurs (4).
- Blue: health hazard
- Red: fire hazard
- White: other hazard

43. B: If a patient has undergone bilateral mastectomies with surgeries 5 years apart, the phlebotomist should ask the physician for instructions regarding the appropriate site. If policy precludes the use of the lower extremities, the venipuncture site is usually the arm on the side with the most distant mastectomy because the healing is more advanced. However, placing a tourniquet on the side of the mastectomy increases the risk of lymphedema, and the impaired lymphatic filtering and drainage also increases the risk of infection.

44. D: The factor that is likely to have the greatest effect on the CBC (complete blood count) is dehydration because it decreases the fluid portion of the blood, resulting in hemoconcentration. This causes the relative RBC count to increase, as well as the hematocrit. Aerobic exercise has been shown to decrease WBC and neutrophil counts. Environmental temperature may alter some values in a CBC (RBC, Hct, MCV MCH and MCHC) if the sample is stored at room temperature for extended periods of time (≥24 hours).

45. C: When collecting a blood specimen from an ambulatory patient in the home environment, the patient should be placed recumbent or in a chair with arm supports. Venipuncture should never be carried out with the patient sitting in a chair without arm rests because, if the patient faints, the patient could easily fall out of the chair and suffer injuries. If no chair with arms is available, blood can be drawn with the patient lying in bed or on a sofa.

46. A: If venipuncture is done on the basilic vein and the blood returns bright red and pulsing, this indicates accidental arterial draw. Venous blood should be dark purplish red, not bright red, which indicates oxygenated blood. Pulsing is characteristic of arterial blood. The basilic vein lies very close to the brachial artery. The most common reason for accidental arterial draw is deep probing for a vein. Hematoma and compression of the nerves, sometimes resulting in permanent injury, can occur if the arterial draw is not identified and adequate pressure applied to stop bleeding.

47. C: The phlebotomist should observe a venipuncture site for at least 5–10 seconds for signs of excessive or persistent bleeding before applying a gauze pressure bandage. If there is bleeding, then direct pressure should be applied until the bleeding is stopped and then the pressure dressing is applied. The patient should avoid exposing the site to direct pressure (purse strap, other bag) or exertion for the next several hours to avoid reopening the wound and causing bleeding.

48. B: If a patient has severely impaired circulation in the legs and has had a recent bilateral mastectomy, the best choice for a blood draw is probably an artery. Blood cannot be drawn from the foot or ankle veins if the circulation is impaired, and blood should not be drawn from a vein on the side of a mastectomy, which (in this case) is bilateral, because the circulation may be impaired and edema may be present. An arterial blood draw is outside of the scope of practice of the phlebotomist.

49. D: The type of blood cell that does not contain a nucleus is the platelet, which is not formed as a distinct cell (as are other blood cells) but rather is a product of the destruction of another cell. Large cells called megakaryocytes proliferate in the red bone marrow. These cells fragment into many small particles, the platelets, so these particles are not complete cells. The platelets are about half the size of erythrocytes (red blood cells) and survive about 10 days.

50. D: Cortisol is a test that requires a timed specimen. Because cortisol levels vary during the day, the blood for the test is usually drawn first thing in the morning. In some cases, patients are administered 1 mg of dexamethasone the night before the test. Patients are typically asked to avoid strenuous exercise for 24 hours before the test, and some medications may be held that can affect the test results, including anticonvulsants, estrogens, synthetic steroids, and androgens.

51. C: Safety features for venipuncture needles may not be detachable but rather must be a permanent integral part of the needle. The safety feature must ensure that the hands stay behind the needle and must be activated by one hand only. The safety feature should be easy to use and remain in place when the needle is discarded. Safety features may sheath, blunt, or retract the needle after use, depending on the manufacturer.

52. A: If a patient had a right mastectomy 6 months previously, blood may be drawn from the left arm. Blood generally should not be obtained on the side of a mastectomy, regardless of the length of time since surgery. Any degree of lymphedema may alter the results of the blood tests, and the patient is at increased risk of infection from venipuncture. If no other site is available, then a physician's order should be obtained regarding use of this site before attempting to withdraw blood from the side of the mastectomy.

53. D: When doing a venipuncture on a patient under investigation (PUI) for Ebola or with confirmed Ebola, the phlebotomist must use a combination of standard, contact, and droplet isolation plus enhanced measures because of the high risk of becoming infected with any contact with the patient's body fluids, including perspiration and droplets transmitted through coughing. The phlebotomist must follow Ebola protocols exactly, donning and removing PPE under direct supervision to ensure each step is carried out correctly.

54. C: At room temperature (20 °C to 25 °C [68 °F–77 °F]), complete clotting usually occurs within 30–60 minutes. Chilling the specimen will delay the clotting time, and the clotting time will be prolonged in patients who are receiving anticoagulants. Some collection devices contain activators to speed up the clotting time if the sample must be tested quickly. For example, thrombin results in coagulation within 5 minutes and glass/silica particles within 15–30 minutes.

55. C: RBCs (red blood cells) normally circulate in the bloodstream for 120 days, although this duration may be decreased with some diseases, such as sickle cell disease. During the normal 120-day lifespan, an RBC travels throughout the body approximately 75,000 times. While many old cells are destroyed in the liver and spleen by macrophages and excreted daily, production normally keeps pace so that a stable number of RBCs continues to circulate.

56. D: During a venipuncture, if the patient cries out and complains of severe pain, the most appropriate response is to immediately remove the needle even if it is in the middle of a draw. Severe pain may be an indication of damage to a nerve. Symptoms of nerve injury may additionally include shooting pain or shock-like electrical pain, tingling, numbness, or tremor in the limb. If the blood draw must still be done, another site (such as the opposite arm) must be selected. The injury must be documented, and the ordering health-care provider must be notified.

57. C: Blood from infants under one year of age is collected by heel stick (lateral areas), as the child's veins are generally too small for venipuncture. Once a site is selected, it should be thoroughly cleansed with antiseptic (usually 70% isopropyl alcohol) and air-dried completely. The best choice of lancet is an automated one with a controlled length of lancet to ensure it does not insert more than 2 mm, which may result in damage to the bone.

58. B: Whether the needlestick is to the patient or the phlebotomist, the needlestick protocol should be followed because, even though the needle may the patient's own blood, it may also inject bacteria found on the surface of the skin when it accidentally sticks the patient. The area should be washed with soap and water, and bandaged as necessary. The incident should be reported to a supervisor and an incident report filed to ensure that the patient receives proper medical attention and observation.

59. A: If a patient with rheumatoid arthritis has severe flexion contractures of both arms and hands, the best solution for selecting a venipuncture site is probably to ask the patient, who likely has had experience with blood draws and knows which sites are most easily accessed. A winged infusion set with 12-inch tubing may be the best choice because it allows for more flexibility in accessing veins when the patient is unable to extend or rotate a limb.

60. D: If a sample is designated as QNS, this means that the quantity is not sufficient for the test that has been ordered. In this case, the sample is rejected and another sample must be obtained. QNS is a common reason for rejecting chemistry specimens. The phlebotomist should review requirements for tests to ensure that the volume of the specimen is adequate. Reasons for QNS may include using expired tubes (resulting in decreased vacuum) and not ensuring complete filling of the tube before changing tubes. QNS may also occur if a patient has difficult-to-access veins.

61. B: After collecting a blood sample, a tube containing sodium citrate as an additive should be inverted 3–4 times rather than the 5–10 times required of other additives. Sodium citrate is an anticoagulant that binds to calcium, preventing blood clotting. Sodium citrate is preferred for coagulation tests (partial thromboplastin time [PTT] and activated partial thromboplastin time [aPTT]) because it best preserves coagulation factors. Tubes that contain sodium citrate have light-blue colored stoppers or black stoppers in special tubes used for the erythrocyte sedimentation rate. Shaking or inverting too much may activate the platelets, resulting in a shortened coagulation time.

62. C: Peak levels of cortisol are usually obtained in the early morning as there is a predictable diurnal variation in blood levels. The lowest level is usually around midnight. Exercise increases cortisol levels. Because of the diurnal variation, multiple tests of cortisol levels are often done (such as at 8 AM, 4PM) in order to evaluate the changes in levels. The total cortisol level—which is obtained with a 24-hour urine—does not show this variation. With abnormal findings, additional testing, such as dexamethasone suppression and ACTH stimulation, is often done.

63. A: If a patient sitting in a chair has a generalized convulsive seizure during venipuncture, the appropriate response is to discontinue venipuncture and call for help to ease the patient to the floor in order to avoid patient injury. The patient should be placed on one side if possible, but movements should not be restrained, and nothing should be placed in the patient's mouth. If possible, a pillow or blanket should be placed under the patient's head and restrictive clothing should be loosened. The time that the seizure begins and ends should be noted and first-aid personnel should be notified.

64. B: While wearing gloves and using care not to allow the collection tube to come into contact with any items on the blood collection tray, the phlebotomist should carefully wipe all blood from the collection tube with a disinfectant and then seal the collection tube in a biohazard bag prior to placing it on the blood collection tray for transport to the laboratory. The gloves should be disposed of in the hazardous waste container.

65. B: When collecting a specimen from a patient in a long-term-care facility, the first thing that the phlebotomist should do is to check in at the nursing station. The phlebotomist needs to ask for information about any special concerns regarding the patient, such as the need for assistance if the patient is confused or any type of restriction that applies to the patient. As always, the phlebotomist should always knock on the door or announce his or her arrival before entering the room and explain the purpose of the visit.

66. B: When using a portable heat block to maintain a blood specimen at body temperature, the phlebotomist should expect the heat block to hold the temperature for approximately 15 minutes. Typically, the specimen tube should also be prewarmed to body temperature (37 °C [98.6 °F]). The specimens should be transported to the lab as soon as possible and transferred to a heating device that will maintain the appropriate temperature.

67. D: Control runs of automated systems should be carried out at the beginning of each day to ensure that the equipment is fully operational. Automated systems carry out laboratory tests with little input from personnel once the equipment is loaded with the appropriate samples. Automated systems may produce errors; therefore, close monitoring is essential. Routine maintenance should be carried out on a scheduled basis. Maintenance may include cleaning spills, changing reagents, discarding waste, changing parts as needed, and making adjustments.

68. B: Serum specimens can be centrifuged after clotting is completed. All specimens for tests carried out on serum or plasma must be centrifuged to separate the liquid from the cellular portions of the blood. However, plasma specimens that are collected in tubes with anticoagulant can be centrifuged immediately. It is important to avoid recentrifugation because this may result in hemolysis and can alter the testing results.

69. A: Phlebotomists are especially at risk for developing an allergic response to latex because it is commonly used in tourniquets, gloves, and other medical equipment and devices, such as blood pressure cuffs. Powdered latex gloves increase risk because the proteins in the latex adhere to the powder particles. Contact dermatitis is frequently the first indication of an allergic response, but reactions can be severe, including anaphylaxis. Because some patients are also sensitive to latex, non-latex gloves and tourniquets should be used whenever possible.

70. D: For most POC pregnancy tests, the earliest time to take the test for accuracy is 1 day after a missed period. If the patient is unsure about when her period is due, then the test can be taken 21 days after unprotected sex. Some newer tests are now able to detect pregnancy even before a missed period. However, testing too early can sometimes produce a false negative, so tests taken after a missed period are usually more accurate. Testing is carried out with a urine sample.

71. B: The total blood volume of a child is approximately 75–80 mL/kg. The volume is greater in a premature neonate, ranging from 89 to approximately 105 mL/kg. The volume of blood in a full-term neonate ranges from 82-86 mL/kg. The volume peaks at approximately 4 weeks and then decreases over the next few months. The total volume of blood in the adult typically ranges from 65-70 mL/kg.

72. C: With rapid influenza diagnostic tests (RIDTS), positive or negative test results are more likely to be accurate if the sample is obtained within 4 days of the onset of symptoms. Both false negatives and false positives may occur, although false negatives are more common than false positives. Various tests are available. Some differentiate between influenza A and B, and others do not. Different types of specimens (nasal, throat swab) are required, depending on the manufacturer.

73. D: When decanting a 24-hour urine specimen, which may splash, into a sink to a sanitary sewer, the phlebotomist should wear facial protection and a fluid-proof apron in addition to the standard personal protective equipment (PPE) (gloves, lab coat). The phlebotomist should stand close to the sink and pour close to the sink opening. Water should not be running while decanting because this increases the risk of splashing, but copious amounts of water should be run after the decanting is completed.

74. C: The antiseptic that is most commonly used for cleaning the venipuncture site is isopropyl alcohol 70%, which is more effective at destroying pathogens than 90% isopropyl alcohol. Povidone-iodine may also be used and is generally used for blood alcohol testing, but it must be removed from the skin after the venipuncture. Chlorhexidine gluconate may be used as an antiseptic also and is sometimes mixed with 67% isopropyl alcohol.

75. B: The maximum number of samples or tests that can be performed each hour by an assay system is the throughput. The throughput is calculated keeping the required dwell times in mind. The throughput varies from one type of equipment to another. Throughput is one of the aspects to consider when determining turnaround time for a laboratory. Turnaround time is a key element of quality control performance. Generally, the turnaround time for the most common laboratory tests should be less than 60 minutes.

76. D: The additive that is most effective at preserving coagulation factors is sodium citrate. Light blue–capped evacuated collection tubes contain sodium citrate and are used for coagulation tests, which are conducted on plasma. The volume ratio of blood to anticoagulant must be 9:1 to obtain the correct clotting times, so the tubes must be filled to capacity, and overfilling and underfilling must be avoided. The collection tubes must be inverted immediately to prevent activation of clotting, but shaking or mixing vigorously must be avoided because it may activate platelets and decrease clotting times.

77. B: For therapeutic drug monitoring, the peak time for most drugs after intramuscular injection is approximately 60 minutes whereas the peak time after IV administration is approximately 30 minutes. Oral medications, on the other hand, usually peak after 1-2 hours. Peak levels are assessed to ensure that the patient is not receiving a toxic dose of medication. Medications that are assessed with therapeutic drug monitoring typically have a narrow therapeutic range.

78. A: If a patient reports a history of episodes of syncope, the most appropriate response is to place the patient in a recumbent position, either lying flat or reclining in a chair, so that he or she does not fall or experience injury if an episode of syncope occurs. Syncope is an episode of fainting that occurs with a sudden drop in blood pressure, sometimes associated with stress or fear.

Patients who are fearful of needles or the sight of blood are especially at risk for syncope during venipuncture.

79. D: Strenuous exercise may increase values of lactic dehydrogenase (LD) and creatinine phosphokinase (CK) for more than 24 hours after exercise stops. Even mild exercise may increase some laboratory values for a short period of time but these changes dissipate so quickly that they rarely affect findings. Short-term changes may occur after exercise with lactic acid, protein, creatinine, and some enzymes. The degree to which exercise affects laboratory values depends on the type of exercise and the duration that elapses between exercise and testing.

80. A: When peritoneal fluid is aspirated during a paracentesis and must be tested for cell counts, the type of specimen tube that is indicated is EDTA. A sterile heparinized tube is used for cultures, a heparin or sodium fluoride tube is for chemistries, and a nonanticoagulant tube is for biochemical tests. Serous fluid is usually pale yellow in appearance and may include pericardial fluid that surrounds the heart, pleural fluid from the space around the lungs, and peritoneal fluid from the abdominal cavity.

81. A: If the phlebotomist tells a friend about doing a venipuncture for a famous actor who is hospitalized, this constitutes a Health Insurance Portability and Accountability Act of 1996 (HIPAA) violation. No protected health information, including the fact that the person was hospitalized or having tests, can be divulged without written authorization. In fact, this information must not be shared with coworkers either unless they are involved in the patient's care and have a need to know.

82. B: If a patient must do a 72-hour stool collection for fecal fat analysis, the stool should be kept under refrigeration during the collection period. The patient is provided a large gallon container with a lid and written and verbal instructions. The patient should be cautioned to avoid contaminating the stool specimen with urine, which may alter the test results. One method of collecting the stool is to place plastic wrap securely over the back half of the toilet bowl. Special collection devices are also available.

83. D: Cerebrospinal fluid (CSF) is usually collected in three or four numbered tubes. If four tubes are collected, they are tested in the following manner:

1. Chemistry and immunology tests
2. Microbiology studies
3. Cell count and differential
4. Cytology and special tests

The cell count is conducted with the third tube that is collected because the first two tubes are more likely to be contaminated with blood cells that were introduced during the spinal tap.

84. C: Blood type is determined by the presence or absence of antigens on the red blood cells (RBCs). If a person's blood is type A, A antigens are on the RBCs, and the plasma agglutinin (antibody) that is present in the person's blood is anti-B. Type B blood has B antigens on the RBCs and anti-A agglutinins in the plasma. Type O blood has no antigens on the RBCs but anti-A and anti-B agglutinins in the plasma. Individuals with type O blood, specifically O-negative blood, are considered universal donors due to their lack of antigens, making the blood less likely to be rejected or result in a transfusion reaction.

85. D: When venipuncture is done in edematous tissue, the results will likely be altered because the sample may contain tissue fluid. Additionally, veins are often harder to locate in edematous tissue, and bleeding may persist longer than usual. Edematous tissue is more prone to injury from the tourniquet because the tissue is stretched. Whenever possible, a nonedematous site should be used for venipuncture. If the edema is because an IV has infiltrated, the phlebotomist must notify the nurse immediately.

86. D: Black-capped collection tubes are used only for ESR (erythrocyte sedimentation rate). These tubes contain sodium citrate as an additive. The ESR measures the rate at which red blood cells fall to the bottom of the collection tube within an hour. The more that fall, the higher the sedimentation rate. The ESR is a non-specific test that indicates an inflammatory process is occurring. Proteins that are produced in response to infection, cancer, or some autoimmune diseases promote clumping of the red blood cells, increasing the rate at which they fall.

87. D: If category B infectious materials must be transported out of the area for testing, specimens must not exceed 500 mL or 500 g. The sample must be triple wrapped with the inner container being watertight and with a screw-on cap. This container must be wrapped in absorbent material and placed in a leakproof bag, which is then placed in a third outer container made of rigid material (wood, metal, plastic, or corrugated fiberboard). The outer container must be leakproof if ice is used. Ice or dry ice is placed about the secondary container.

88. C: The pattern of antecubital veins that is predominant in most populations is the H pattern. The veins that are most prominent in the H pattern include the cephalic, median cubital, and basilic veins. The veins that are most prominent in the M pattern include the cephalic, median cephalic, median basilic, and basilic veins. Although these two patterns are common, some patients have atypical patterns of veins rather than the H or M configuration.

89. C: When conducting the urine dipstick test, the dipstick should be dipped into the urine and then withdrawn and tapped lightly on the side of the container to remove excess urine. Then, the dipstick should be held in a horizontal position so that the urine on the dipstick pools and stays in touch with the reagents for the specified time period, usually ranging from 30 seconds to 2 minutes, depending on the type of dipstick. Then, the dipstick is compared with a color chart to determine the results.

90. D: When obtaining a blood specimen for coagulation tests (PT, aPTT), the use of a discard tube is indicated when a winged (butterfly) blood collection set is used and the coagulation tube is filled first. At one time, it was standard procedure to obtain a discard tube of 5 mL of blood when the coagulation tube was the first tube to be filled, but studies have indicated that this is not necessary. However, when using a winged (butterfly) needle, the discard tube is collected in order to prime the tubing so that the correct ratio of blood to anticoagulant is maintained.

91. A: Collecting a specimen from a vascular access device (VAD) may result in hemolysis of a specimen. A specimen should also not be collected during an intravenous (IV) line start. Additional precautions include ensuring that the needle is secure, avoiding forcibly pulling on a plunger to withdraw blood or forcefully transferring blood from a syringe into a tube, discontinuing a sluggish draw, avoiding the use of 25-gauge needles, limiting tourniquet use to 60 seconds, and avoiding shaking or vigorously mixing specimens.

92. A: If a blood specimen is to be obtained for the trough (lowest blood concentration) level of a drug, the best time to draw the blood is usually 15 minutes before the next scheduled dose because the concentration should be at its lowest point. Trough levels may be checked to ensure that a minimum amount of drug remains in the blood. The levels may also be used to determine the correct dose and spacing of doses and to help determine the rate of drug absorption.

93. C: When doing a venipuncture, the correct angle of insertion of the needle is usually 30 degrees, per CLSI guidelines. If the angle is too narrow (10-20 degrees), then the needle may not penetrate the vein but may enter only the subcutaneous tissue. If the angle is too steep (>30 degrees), then the needle may go through the vein. However, each patient should be individually assessed. If a patient is extremely thin or is obese, the angle may need to be adjusted slightly to compensate.

94. C: If blood is withdrawn for coagulation studies from a VAD, this requires flushing the VAD lock with preservative-free normal saline (NS) (5–10 mL) and drawing a discard tube first, equal to two times the dead space. For most central lines, 5 mL is adequate as the discard volume, although this may vary so the discard volume needed should always be verified. For coagulation studies, typically a discard volume of six times the dead space is recommended, although if drawing blood from a saline lock, a discard volume of two times the dead space is adequate. After the specimen is obtained, the VAD is again flushed with 5–10 mL of preservative-free NS.

95. A: The most abundant electrolytes in plasma are sodium and chloride (which are used in normal saline). Electrolytes are absorbed into the circulatory system from the intestines or produced as by-products of cellular metabolism. The most important electrolytes are sodium, chloride, potassium, calcium, sulfate, bicarbonate, and hydrogen ions. Electrolytes are excreted through perspiration, urine, and feces. Most electrolytes are maintained in balance as people respond to hunger and thirst.

96. B: Lymph fluid is similar in composition to plasma. As the blood goes through the capillaries, oxygen, water, and other nutrients diffuse through the capillary walls into the tissues. Some of the fluid diffuses back into the capillaries along with waste products, but some of the remaining fluid collects in lymphatic capillaries, where it is referred to as lymph fluid, which is about 95% water. The lymph fluid flows into large lymphatic vessels, which have valves similar to veins so that the fluid moves forward with muscle contractions.

97. C: Tests that are not appropriate for delivery to the lab by pneumatic tube include those in which damage to the cell membrane may affect the test results, such as lactate dehydrogenase, potassium, hemoglobin (plasma), and acid phosphatase. Additionally, samples that must be kept at body temperature, such as cryoglobulins and cold agglutinins, should not be transported by pneumatic tube. Pneumatic tubes are one of the most common methods used to transport specimens to laboratories.

98. C: If a phlebotomist develops dermatitis from all types of gloves, the best solution is to wear glove liners or apply a barrier hand cream specifically designed to prevent irritation from gloves. Continuing to wear gloves, even for brief periods of time, may cause further irritation, which increases the risk of infection for both the phlebotomist and the patients. Additionally, if the hands are irritated, cleansing with alcohol-based rubs or soap and water may increase irritation.

99. D: If the safety device on the venipuncture needle fails to activate, leaving the needle exposed, in order to dispose of the needle, the phlebotomist should carefully place the needle and attached tube holder in the sharps container. Needles should never be bent, broken, recapped, or wrapped, as these actions may result in needlestick injuries. The phlebotomist should report the failure of the safety device to a supervisor so that other needle supplies can be evaluated.

100. C: If less than the recommended volume necessary for blood cultures is obtained, the aerobic specimen tube should be filled completely first and then the remainder is placed in the anaerobic tube. The tubes should be inverted gently a few times to prevent clotting. The only anticoagulant that is acceptable for blood cultures is sodium polyanetholesulfonate (SPS), and the blood can be collected directly into tubes with SPS and then transferred to the medium for culture.

101. B: All laboratory testing in the United States, except for research testing, is regulated by the Centers for Medicare & Medicaid Services (CMS) through CLIA, which is implemented through the Division of Laboratory Services and serves approximately 244,000 laboratories. Laboratories receiving reimbursement from CMS must meet CLIA standards, which ensure that laboratory testing will be accurate and that procedures are followed properly.

102. B: The maximum volume of blood that may be drawn from a 20 lb infant in an eight-week period is approximately 60 mL. CLSI regulations recommend no more than 10% of total blood volume to be drawn from a pediatric patient over an eight-week period. Using the 65-70 mL/kg conversion recommended by the CLSI, this patient's total volume can be calculated as follows:

$$20 \text{ lb} \times \frac{1 \text{ kg}}{2.2 \text{ lb}} = 9.1 \text{ kg}$$

$$9.1 \text{ kg} \times 65 \frac{mL}{kg} = 592 \text{ mL}; 9.1 \text{ kg} \times 70 \frac{mL}{kg} = 637 \text{ mL}$$

So the allowable amount of blood to be drawn in this timeframe is 59-64 mL.

103. D: The specimen for a lactic acid test must be chilled. Other tests that require a chilled specimen include catecholamines, ammonia, pyruvate, adrenocorticotropic hormone, parathyroid hormone, metanephrines (plasma), and gastrin. Chilling the specimen slows the cell metabolism that otherwise continues and protects analytes that are altered by heat. Most specimens that require chilling are chilled in an ice-and-water slurry. A few specimens, such as homocysteine in the gel tube, are chilled on a cooler rack.

104. D: "DNR" means "do not resuscitate" ("no code"). When patients are admitted to the hospital, they are now usually asked if they want to be resuscitated in the event of a cardiac arrest or cessation of breathing. If patients indicate that they do not want resuscitation, then the DNR order is entered into the records so that appropriate health care providers are aware of the patients' wishes. If no DNR order is present, then extraordinary means, such as intubation and ventilation, may be done to sustain life.

105. C: At room temperature, EDTA specimens for erythrocyte sedimentation rate (ESR) must be tested within 4 hours or within 12 hours if the specimen is refrigerated. The ESR is used to diagnose acute infection or inflammatory processes in disease. The test is typically performed on whole blood collected in a lavender/purple EDTA tube. The test determines how quickly RBCs/erythrocytes settle to the bottom of the specimen tube. Inflammation or infection tends to speed this process.

106. D: Mouth pipetting, sucking a laboratory specimen into an open-ended tube, was once common practice in laboratories, but the practice was generally stopped in the 1970s when mechanical pipettes became available. However, mouth pipetting is still commonly used in developing nations where medical supplies are scarce and equipment is often outdated, so phlebotomists who work overseas should be aware that the practice puts them at high risk of disease and should never be utilized.

107. B: The POC test that is most accurate for monitoring heparin therapy is activated clotting time (ACT). Automated ACT analyzers measure how long it takes a blood sample to clot when activators

119

are added to activate the clotting factors. This helps to determine how the body will respond to heparin and is more accurate than aPTT, especially if the patient is receiving high doses of heparin. The normal value for ACT may vary according to the equipment used, but it generally ranges from 70-120 seconds. The therapeutic value generally ranges from 150-600 seconds.

108. C: Warning signs, such as "fall precautions," are usually placed on the patient's door. The phlebotomist should always check the outside of the door for guidance. Other signs include isolation notices or signs indicating limited visitation. If a patient has a severe allergy (such as to latex), this may also be indicated by a sign on the door. In some institutions, pictures are used instead of words for privacy reasons, so the phlebotomist should be familiar with the usual signs.

109. D: The nerve most often injured with venipuncture is the median nerve because blood draws are most frequently done in the antecubital space and the median nerve, which is the largest in the arm, passes through this area. The second most common injury is of the radial nerve, which runs near the cephalic vein on the radial side of the wrist and into the palm of the hand. Venipuncture should be avoided in the 7.5 cm area above the thumb.

110. A: When collecting a capillary blood sample after a fingerstick or heelstick, it is necessary to wipe away the first drop with a gauze pad because this first drop is likely contaminated and may contain some alcohol from the antiseptic, which may cause hemolysis or prevent the blood from forming drops. However, some point-of-care (POC) testing devices, such as those for glucose testing, recommend using the first drop, making it an exception.

111. D: If the needle hits the median nerve during an antecubital venipuncture, the most common patient complaint is severe shock-like pain. If this occurs, the initial response should be to immediately remove the needle and apply pressure because continuing with the venipuncture may result in permanent damage to the nerve. Usually the pain resolves within a few hours, but if the nerve is damaged, the patient may develop permanent pain and weakness, including complex regional pain syndrome.

112. D: The platelet function test is used to determine a patient's response to aspirin therapy or other antiplatelet therapies. This test is also used to assess a patient's response to medications before cardiac catheterization or surgery. Platelet function tests can help clinicians assess and predict the risk of bleeding and of thrombosis associated with platelet dysfunction before, during, and after the procedures.

113. B: Gloves should generally be donned prior to cleansing the skin, although with concerns about infection, they may be donned earlier. For example, for COVID-19 precautions, gloves are typically worn for all patient contact. However, the usual procedure is to apply the tourniquet, palpate and select the vein, select the needed supplies, and then don gloves before cleansing the site and carrying out the venipuncture.

114. C: A blood specimen for a CBC should be collected in a tube that contains Na_2EDTA (an anticoagulant). The CBC is done on whole blood. The evacuated collection tube is lavender-capped and should be inverted at least 8 times after the specimen is collected to ensure that the sample is adequately anticoagulated because even small clots render the specimen unusable. The CBC includes Hgb (hemoglobin), Hct (hematocrit), RBC, RBC indices, WBC and differential, and platelet count.

115. A: Hemostasis refers to stoppage of bleeding when vessels have been damaged or torn. Hemostasis helps to prevent blood loss through three mechanisms:

- Vasospasm: Damaging a blood vessel causes the smooth muscles to contract, effectively sealing off small tears. This reaction persists for 30 minutes.
- Platelet plug: Platelets adhere to damaged vessels, especially the collagen in connective tissue that underlies the endothelial lining of vessels. Collagen causes the platelets to change shape and adhere to each other, creating a clot to block bleeding.
- Coagulation of blood: Release of biochemicals triggers both intrinsic and extrinsic clotting mechanisms.

116. B: If, after leaving a patient's room, the phlebotomist is asked by the patient's brother what tests the patient is having, the phlebotomist should provide no information. Under the federal Health Insurance Portability and Accountability Act (HIPAA), healthcare providers are prohibited from violating an individual's privacy by providing any information about the patient without the explicit permission of the patient. The exception is if the patient is a minor and information is provided to a parent or legal guardian or the person asking for information has power of attorney for healthcare.

117. C: When the phlebotomist enters an isolation room to draw blood, the phlebotomy tray should be left in a secure place outside of the room where unauthorized people cannot gain access to it. The phlebotomist should carry only equipment needed for the sample collection into the room, following procedures for use of PPE and the type of isolation. All of the items taken into the room should be discarded inside the room in appropriate containers except for the tubes of blood, which should be sealed in a leak-proof plastic bag for transport.

118. B: The test specimen for bilirubin is photosensitive and must be protected from exposure to light (artificial or natural) by wrapping the specimen container in aluminum foil, using an amber specimen container, or placing the specimen in a biohazard bag or other container that blocks light. Bilirubin may decrease by half after an hour of exposure to light, especially specimens obtained from capillaries because they are exposed to light during collection. Other specimens that are photosensitive include beta-carotene, folate, vitamin A, vitamin B2, vitamin B6, vitamin C, urine porphobilinogen, and urine porphyrins.

119. B: If a patient has made a fist for venipuncture, the point at which he or she should generally be instructed to open the hand is when blood flow is established. The purpose of making a fist is to increase the pressure in the veins and their visibility. The patient should be cautioned to avoid pumping the fist, which can increase potassium levels. The hand may remain clenched during collection if the vein appears that it may collapse if the fist is unclenched.

120. D: When having trouble visualizing a vein, the best approach is to ask the patient to make a fist but to avoid having him or her pump the fist because this may result in hemoconcentration and can affect the test results, especially that of potassium. The fist should be released as soon as blood begins to flow into the collection tube. Vigorously massaging the vein or leaving the tourniquet in place for more than 60 seconds can also cause hemoconcentration.

NHA Phlebotomy Practice Test #2

1. If blood must be drawn from an arm with an IV in place, the phlebotomist should _____.

    a. turn off the IV and wait at least 2 minutes before attempting venipuncture

    b. ask the nurse to turn off the IV and wait 2 minutes before attempting venipuncture

    c. place a tourniquet proximal to the IV and carry out venipuncture distal to the IV

    d. place a tourniquet proximal to the IV and carry out venipuncture proximal to the IV

2. The closure cap of the collection tube that contains sodium citrate is _____.

    a. gray

    b. lavender

    c. green

    d. light blue

3. If the phlebotomist observes another worker placing needles and syringes into a personal bag before leaving work, the best response is to _____.

    a. confront the worker

    b. remain quiet

    c. call the police

    d. notify a supervisor

4. The preferred capillary puncture site for adults and children older than 1 year of age is the _____.

    a. lateral heel

    b. distal segment of the nondominant third or fourth finger

    c. distal segment of the dominant third or fourth finger

    d. earlobe

5. The chain of custody for a blood specimen, such as one for drug testing, begins with the _____.

    a. order

    b. initial patient contact

    c. transfer to the lab

    d. processing

6. Which of the following is a health hazard as opposed to a physical hazard?

    a. Compressed gas

    b. Combustible liquid

    c. Explosive material

    d. Corrosive chemical

7. A test request should include the following specific information about the patient: _____.

    a. name, identification (ID)/record number, gender, and date of birth

    b. name, date of birth, and address

    c. gender, ID/record number, indication for the test, and date of birth

    d. name, ID/record number, telephone number, and date of birth

8. Which one of the following billing codes is used for laboratory testing for inpatients?

    a. ICD-11.
    b. ICD-10-PCS.
    c. ICD-10-CM.
    d. CPT.

9. According to the ADA, to ensure accessibility to patients on crutches or in wheelchairs, at least one space next to the phlebotomy chair must have a minimum area of _____.

    a. 20 × 30 inches
    b. 30 × 48 inches
    c. 36 × 60 inches
    d. 48 × 72 inches

10. If a patient is very angry and yells that the lab tests are a "waste of time," which of the following is the best initial response?

    a. Stay calm and listen
    b. Explain the purpose
    c. Leave the room
    d. Ask the patient to be civil

11. A blood sample in a gray-capped evacuated collection tube should be inverted a minimum of _____.

    a. 5 times
    b. 6 times
    c. 8 times
    d. 12 times

12. If protocol for blood C&S requires skin antisepsis with alcohol (isopropyl 70%) followed by tincture of iodine (2%), but the patient is allergic to iodine, an acceptable alternate procedure is _____.

    a. Wash with soap and water and cleanse once with alcohol
    b. Cleanse twice with alcohol
    c. Cleanse 3 times with alcohol
    d. Wash with soap and water and cleanse twice with alcohol

13. Which of the following is a method of preventing reflux?

    a. Allow back and forth movement in the tube while filling
    b. Maintain the arm in a downward position while filling the tube
    c. Maintain the arm in an upward position while filling the tube
    d. Hold the collection tube very still while filling

14. The order of the draw is determined by the _____.

    a. FDA
    b. CAP
    c. JCAHO
    d. CLSI

15. When conducting a fingerstick glucose test, to transfer the blood from the finger to the test strip, the phlebotomist should _____.
- a. hold the edge of the strip next to the drop of blood
- b. dip the strip directly into the drop of blood
- c. wipe the strip across the drop of blood
- d. use a disposable pipette for transfer

16. When asked to collect blood from a peripheral vascular access device, the phlebotomist should recognize that this procedure_____.
- a. is outside his or her scope of practice
- b. requires supervision
- c. requires additional training
- d. is contraindicated

17. If a patient's test request requires a chemistry panel, a CBC, a PT, and blood typing, in what order should the specimens be drawn, first to last?
- a. CBC, chemistry panel, PT, blood typing.
- b. Chemistry panel, PT, blood typing, CBC.
- c. PT, blood typing, CBC, chemistry panel.
- d. PT, chemistry panel, blood typing, and CBC.

18. With double-pointed needles, the rubber sheath that covers the shorter needle is intended to _____.
- a. prevent needlestick injuries
- b. prevent leakage of blood
- c. indicate the side used for venipuncture
- d. prevent breakage of the needle

19. If an indwelling line, such as a central venous catheter is used to obtain a blood sample, how much blood should be discarded before the sample is collected?
- a. One mL
- b. Two mL
- c. Four mL
- d. Five mL

20. Which one of the following tests CANNOT be carried out on a specimen obtained through heelstick and a capillary blood sample?
- a. CBC.
- b. Glucose (bedside).
- c. Blood gas analysis.
- d. Blood cultures.

21. Using a foot vein for a blood draw _____.
- a. Is prohibited
- b. Poses no increased risks
- c. Increases risk of blood clots
- d. Is negligent

22. If a phlebotomist sustains a needlestick injury, the first step is to _____.

   a. notify the supervisor.
   b. cleanse the puncture site with alcohol-based hand rub
   c. wash the puncture site with soap and water
   d. milk the wound to promote bleeding

23. Underfilling a green-capped evacuated collection tube may result in _____.

   a. Low test results
   b. Clotting
   c. Cell morphology changes
   d. No adverse effects

24. When doing a venipuncture for a CBC, which stopper color indicates the correct tube?

   a. Lavender/Purple.
   b. Light blue.
   c. Pink.
   d. Green.

25. If a patient has paralysis and lack of sensation in the right arm and hand, the best choice for venipuncture is _____.

   a. any appropriate site on the right arm
   b. the dorsal metacarpal veins on the right hand
   c. any appropriate site on the right or left arm
   d. any appropriate site on the left arm

26. For venipuncture, the vein should be anchored _____.

   a. on the right or left of the puncture site (one finger)
   b. on the right and left of the puncture site (two fingers)
   c. proximal to the puncture site
   d. distal to the puncture site

27. The greatest risk when a tube breaks during centrifugation is _____.

   a. Aerosolization of sample
   b. Lacerations/Puncture wounds
   c. Equipment damage
   d. Electric shock

28. A person with blood type AB+ should receive a transfusion with blood type _____.

   a. A+
   b. B+
   c. AB+
   d. A+, B+, or AB+

29. If the phlebotomist is asked to transport a nonblood specimen, such as a urine sample, to the laboratory for testing, the phlebotomist should _____.

   a. accept the specimen for transport
   b. verify that the sample is labeled correctly
   c. refuse to accept the specimen for transport
   d. check with the laboratory supervisor regarding the transport

30. A vital function of the capillaries is to _____.
   a. control the flow of blood
   b. exchange gases, nutrients, and metabolic by-products
   c. stabilize the blood pressure
   d. secrete substances that prevent the clotting of blood

31. If the phlebotomist is accidently splashed with a highly toxic hazardous chemical, what is the minimum length of time that the affected body part should be flushed with water?
   a. 2 minutes
   b. 5 minutes
   c. 10 minutes
   d. 15 minutes

32. When reviewing orders, the abbreviation for the thyroid hormone triiodothyronine is _____.
   a. T_3
   b. T_4
   c. TSH
   d. TBG

33. When collecting a blood specimen in a collection tube that contains an additive, _____.
   a. the collection tube should be higher than the puncture site
   b. the collection tube should be at the same level as the puncture site
   c. the collection tube should be lower than the puncture site
   d. the collection tube should be at the same level or lower than the puncture site

34. The primary use of non-additive evacuated plastic collection tubes is for _____.
   a. practice tubes
   b. cultures
   c. contaminated samples
   d. discard tubes

35. Which one of the following agencies provides standards for performance and testing of all types of laboratory functions and microbiology?
   a. CLSI.
   b. WHO.
   c. NCQA.
   d. CLIAC.

36. The left atrioventricular valve of the heart is called the _____.
   a. aortic valve
   b. mitral valve
   c. pulmonic valve
   d. tricuspid valve

37. The Joint Commission is primarily a(n) _____.

    a. research facility
    b. regulatory agency
    c. FDA advisory board
    d. accrediting organization.

38. When delivering a blood specimen that requires STAT testing to the laboratory, the phlebotomist must _____.

    a. ensure that the specimen is marked as STAT
    b. place it in a STAT rack
    c. assume that the testing personnel are aware of the STAT request
    d. notify the testing personnel of the STAT request and receive verbal acknowledgement

39. If petechiae are noted on the patient's skin distal to the tourniquet, this suggests that _____.

    a. the tourniquet has been improperly applied
    b. the patient is having an allergic reaction
    c. the patient may have a coagulation defect
    d. the tourniquet has been on for too long

40. The correct method of removing a stopper from a specimen tube is to _____.

    a. twist the stopper off
    b. pull it straight up and away from the tube
    c. pop the stopper off by applying pressure on one side with a thumb
    d. use forceps to grasp the stopper and pull it from the tube

41. Which government agency is responsible for laws governing the use of gloves when carrying out a venipuncture?

    a. USDA
    b. FDA
    c. CDC
    d. OSHA

42. Iatrogenic anemia in a neonate is caused by _____.

    a. Excessive bleeding
    b. Excessive blood draws
    c. Inadequate nutrition
    d. Genetic disease

43. For therapeutic drug monitoring, critical times include _____.

    a. the time of the last dose and the time the specimen was collected
    b. the time of the last dose and the time the specimen was examined
    c. the time the specimen was collected and the time the specimen was examined
    d. the time the specimen was collected

44. Physician office laboratories are most often accredited by _____.

    a. CLIA
    b. COLA
    c. CAP
    d. The Joint Commission

45. When using an evacuated tube system for venipuncture, the phlebotomist can determine that a tube is properly filled when _____.

    a. the vacuum is exhausted
    b. the volume fills to the "full" line
    c. the volume fills the tube completely
    d. the volume appears adequate on examination

46. When using micro-collection tubes for a finger stick, the collection tube that should usually be filled first is _____.

    a. Gray-capped
    b. Lavender-capped
    c. Green-capped
    d. Yellow-capped

47. Which one of the following governmental agencies requires an exposure control plan that outlines methods to reduce staff injury and exposure?

    a. CMS.
    b. OSHA.
    c. TJC.
    d. CDC.

48. The correct collection tube for ethanol level is _____.

    a. Light blue–capped
    b. Royal blue–capped
    c. Gray-capped
    d. Green-capped

49. The primary function of WBCs is to _____.

    a. oxygenate tissue
    b. fight infection
    c. facilitate blood clotting
    d. inhibit blood clotting

50. Which one of the following is NOT a reason to avoid removing stoppers from blood specimen tubes prior in the precentrifugation period?

    a. To prevent a decrease in pH.
    b. To prevent a loss of CO_2.
    c. To prevent concentration of the specimen.
    d. To prevent contamination.

51. For which of the following tests must blood be drawn from an artery?

    a. Anti-hemophilic factor
    b. Chromosome analysis
    c. Hemoglobin A1c
    d. Blood gases

52. The innermost layer of an artery is the _____.

    a. tunica media
    b. tunica externa
    c. adventitia
    d. endothelium

53. When using a pediatric vein transilluminator with an infant, the transilluminator should be _____.

    a. placed in the palm of the child's hand
    b. held in place over the veins by a second person
    c. placed in a holder above the puncture site
    d. run along the surface of the skin to illuminate the veins

54. When loading a centrifuge that holds multiple tubes, if only one tube needs to be centrifuged, the phlebotomist should _____.

    a. place the single tube in the centrifuge and complete the centrifugation
    b. place the tube and an empty tube across from it in the centrifuge
    c. place the tube and a tube filled with the same volume of water across from it in the centrifuge
    d. wait until another blood sample is available and then centrifuge both

55. For which of the following tests must the blood specimen be maintained at body temperature until processing?

    a. Cold agglutinins
    b. Lactic acid
    c. pH
    d. Parathyroid hormone

56. Which one of the following vein-finder devices projects a pattern map of the veins on the skin?

    a. Ultrasound.
    b. Near-infrared light.
    c. Transilluminator.
    d. Vein-finder glasses.

57. In an inpatient facility, PPE for the phlebotomist must be provided by _____.

    a. the phlebotomist
    b. the employer
    c. the FDA
    d. OSHA

58. When using an evacuated tube system for venipuncture, how can the phlebotomist determine that the needle is correctly positioned in the vein?

a. A flash of blood is seen at the hub.
b. Blood flows into the holder.
c. The needle slightly vibrates.
d. The phlebotomist feels a decrease in resistance.

59. If a coagulation test requires platelet-poor plasma, it is necessary to _____.

a. centrifuge the specimen, remove three-quarters of the plasma into an aliquot tube, and centrifuge the aliquot
b. centrifuge the specimen, let the specimen set for 10 minutes, and centrifuge again
c. centrifuge the specimen at twice the usual duration of time before removing the plasma
d. centrifuge the specimen, remove half of the plasma into an aliquot tube, and centrifuge the specimen again

60. When transporting a specimen at room temperature, an appropriate temperature is _____.

a. 37 °C
b. 34 °C
c. 22 °C
d. 18 °C

61. When opening and aliquoting a specimen, the required PPE includes _____.

a. gloves
b. gown and gloves
c. gown, gloves, N95 respirator, and face shield
d. gown, gloves, and face shield

62. When collecting blood samples in evacuated collection tubes that contain sodium citrate or ACD, the ratio of blood to additive must be _____.

a. 10:1
b. 9:1
c. 8:2
d. 7:3

63. The phlebotomist should evaluate the risk of violence with _____.

a. Confused patients
b. All patients
c. Inebriated patients
d. Angry patients

64. If an elderly patient has rolling veins, which of the following is the best solution?

a. Apply a tourniquet immediately above the venipuncture site
b. Use a winged infusion set with syringe
c. Use a winged infusion set with evacuated tube
d. Anchor the vein with the thumb

65. For venipuncture, which vein should always be selected as the last option?

a. Median cubital.
b. Cephalic.
c. Basilic.
d. Dorsal metacarpal.

66. Which of the following should NOT be disposed of in a sharps container?

a. Blood-stained gauze
b. Tube holder
c. Lancet
d. Opened clean needle

67. Metal filings ("fleas") may be used with capillary blood glass collection tubes to _____.

a. Seal the tube ends
b. Collect the blood sample
c. Conduct the heel stick
d. Mix blood with anticoagulant

68. If a very small hematoma is evident during venipuncture, the best initial response is to _____.

a. remove the needle, elevate the arm, and apply pressure
b. remove the needle and apply an ice compress
c. remove the needle and apply pressure
d. observe and complete the venipuncture

69. Which one of the following steps can help prevent the development of a hematoma?

a. Maintain the position of the needle throughout the specimen collection.
b. Remove the needle before removing the tourniquet.
c. Remove the needle before removing the tube from the holder.
d. Bandage the puncture site immediately after needle removal.

70. If a gray-capped collection tube is overfilled, the result may be _____.

a. no effect
b. low test result
c. high test result
d. clotting of the specimen

71. Sputum specimens should ideally be obtained _____.

a. after 4 hours of fasting
b. first thing in the morning upon arising
c. at any time of day
d. in the evening just before bed

72. Alcohol-based antisepsis is more commonly used than povidone-iodine–based antisepsis because _____.

a. Alcohol is more effective
b. Alcohol is less expensive
c. Povidone-iodine is more irritating to the skin
d. Povidone-iodine is more likely to cause allergic response

73. After birth, RBCs are produced almost exclusively in the _____.

  a. spleen
  b. liver
  c. red bone marrow
  d. yellow bone marrow

74. During venipuncture, if the needle appears to be in the vein but no blood is flowing and a slight vibration or quiver of the needle is noted, the most appropriate initial response is to _____.

  a. immediately discontinue the venipuncture
  b. remove the vacuum tube, pull back slightly on the needle, and reinsert the vacuum tube
  c. rotate the needle slightly to the right or left
  d. remove the vacuum tube, gently insert the needle further, and reinsert the vacuum tube

75. How long after a patient undergoing a C-urea breath test has completed the baseline exhalation sample and swallowed the synthetic urea solution should the second exhalation sample be taken?

  a. 5 minutes.
  b. 10 minutes.
  c. 15 minutes.
  d. 30 minutes.

76. If serum appears milky, this likely indicates _____.

  a. Lipemia
  b. Bacterial infection
  c. Viral infection
  d. Dehydration

77. An electrolyte panel includes _____.

  a. CO_2, Cl, K, and Na
  b. CO_2, Cl, Ca, and K
  c. Cl, K, Na, and PO_4
  d. CO2, PO_4, Na, and K

78. Within a 24-hour period for pediatric or critically ill patients, what percentage of total blood volume can be collected?

  a. 1–2%.
  b. 3–5%.
  c. 6–8%.
  d. 10%.

79. After using a needle and tube holder to collect a blood specimen, the tube holder should be _____.

  a. Separated from the needle for reuse
  b. Separated from the needle for disposal in the hazardous waste container
  c. Disposed of as one unit with the needle in the sharps container
  d. Separated from the needle and disposed of in open waste container

80. What is the purpose of a Vein Entry Indicator Device (VEID)?

a. Indicate when a needle penetrates a vein
b. Identify the pattern of veins
c. Differentiate arteries from veins
d. Prevent hematomas from venipuncture

81. Which one of the following tests should be available on a POC ABG analyzer?

a. PCO_2.
b. Hgb.
c. Na.
d. Hct.

82. Which of the following may violate the chain of custody for a forensic specimen?

a. Signing the chain of custody form
b. Asking a nurse to temporarily store the specimen
c. Placing the specimen in a transfer bag
d. Documenting the patient's identification

83. Which of the 4 stages of hemostasis occurs first?

a. Formation of platelet plug
b. Vasoconstriction
c. Fibrinolysis
d. Formation of fibrin clot

84. If a patient is chewing gum when the phlebotomist arrives to collect a blood specimen, the phlebotomist should _____.

a. ask the patient to stop chewing during the venipuncture
b. ask the patient to remove the gum before proceeding
c. tell the patient to be careful not to swallow the gum
d. ignore the fact that the patient is chewing gum

85. When carrying out POC testing for PT/INR with an analyzer, such as the CoaguChek XS Plus, a capillary blood drop should generally be applied to the test strip or other collection device within _____.

a. 5 seconds
b. 10 seconds
c. 15 seconds
d. 20 seconds

86. Most of the blood in the body is found in the _____.

a. arteries
b. heart
c. lungs
d. veins

87. If blood cannot be obtained from either arm, before a foot or ankle can be used for drawing blood, the phlebotomist should _____.

    a. check with a supervisor
    b. obtain a physician's order
    c. ask the patient's permission
    d. review the procedure

88. Which of the following items requires disinfection?

    a. Surgical instruments
    b. Blood pressure cuffs
    c. Furniture in the waiting area
    d. Windows

89. The primary purpose of therapeutic drug monitoring (TDM) is to _____.

    a. Identify optimal dosing
    b. Determine abuse of drugs
    c. Wean patient off of drugs
    d. Prevent adverse effects

90. If asked to draw blood from a hospitalized patient who has lost her armband, the first action should be to _____.

    a. ask staff to replace the armband
    b. ask the patient for two identifiers
    c. verify the patient's identification with staff
    d. verify the correct room number

91. Which of the following evacuated collection tubes should NOT be used to collect a specimen for a BMP?

    a. Red-capped with clot activator
    b. Red/Black SST
    c. Lavender-capped
    d. Green-capped

92. If a venipuncture is required from an elderly patient with obvious tremors of the upper extremities, the best solution is to _____.

    a. Ask the patient to keep the arm still
    b. Ask a nurse to assist in stabilizing the arm
    c. Use an ankle or foot vein
    d. Refuse to do the venipuncture

93. When carrying out a heelstick blood collection on a newborn, what should be the maximum depth of the puncture?

    a. ≤1 mm.
    b. ≤1.5 mm.
    c. ≤2 mm.
    d. ≤3 mm.

94. If the phlebotomist drops an unused glass collection tube, causing it to break and scatter pieces of glass, the phlebotomist should_____.

    a. Clean up the glass with a wet paper towel
    b. Ask the nursing staff to clean up the glass
    c. Guard the area and notify housekeeping
    d. Notify a supervisor

95. The hydrogen breath test is most often used to test for _____.

    a. *H. pylori* infection
    b. irritable bowel syndrome
    c. small-intestine bacterial overgrowth
    d. lactose intolerance

96. For forensic collection of a blood sample, the specimen container must be _____.

    a. placed and sealed inside a transfer bag
    b. taped shut
    c. personally observed during testing
    d. placed in a clear plastic bag

97. If drawing a blood specimen from an adolescent, the phlebotomist should recognize that most adolescents are _____.

    a. Self-conscious
    b. Belligerent
    c. Fearful
    d. Disinterested

98. In which order should green capped, lavender-capped, and red-capped pediatric micro-collection containers be collected?

    a. Green, lavender, and red
    b. Lavender, green, and red
    c. Red, lavender, and green
    d. Lavender, red, and green

99. Before a blood specimen is collected from a newborn for routine screening for inborn errors of metabolism (IEM), the infant should _____.

    a. Have been nursed or bottle-fed for at least 12 hours
    b. Have been nursed or bottle-fed for at least 24 hours
    c. Avoided nursing or bottle-feeding for at least 2 hours
    d. Avoided nursing or bottle-feeding for at least 4 hours

100. Which of the following equipment is NOT part of that needed for routine venipuncture?

    a. Cotton balls
    b. Gauze sponges
    c. Tube holders
    d. Needles

101. Which of the following is NOT commonly associated with nosocomial infections?

    a. Staphylococcus aureus
    b. Mycobacterium tuberculosis
    c. MRSA
    d. Clostridium difficile

102. Venipuncture of which of the following veins poses the greatest risk of accidental puncture of an artery?

    a. Median cubital vein
    b. Cephalic
    c. Basilic vein
    d. Metacarpal vein

103. The first step in carrying out a venipuncture is to_____.

    a. explain the purpose
    b. obtain consent
    c. identify the patient
    d. identify the site

104. If a patient is very thin with prominent veins that require a low needle angle for venipuncture, the best choice is probably _____.

    a. 21-gauge needle with tube holder
    b. Winged infusion set with syringe
    c. 21-gauge needle with syringe
    d. 23-gauge needle with syringe

105. In the United States, all laboratory testing, except for research, is regulated by _____.

    a. CMS
    b. FDA
    c. CAP
    d. OSHA

106. When doing a blood draw for PT, aPTT, and TT, what is the correct cap color on the collection tube?

    a. Green
    b. Lavender
    c. Light blue
    d. Gray

107. If a venipuncture is requested at a specific time but the phlebotomist mistakenly collects the specimen 30 minutes late, the phlebotomist should _____.

    a. report the late collection immediately
    b. assume that 30 minutes is within an acceptable range of time
    c. write the time of collection on the label
    d. do or say nothing about the late collection unless asked

108. When collecting a capillary blood specimen for bilirubin from a newborn receiving phototherapy for jaundice, it is especially important to _____.

    a. work as quickly as possible
    b. collect the specimen in a clear container
    c. turn off the phototherapy light during collection
    d. avoid blocking the phototherapy lights

109. What percentage of the blood is composed of plasma?

    a. 35%.
    b. 45%.
    c. 55%.
    d. 65%.

110. If the phlebotomist notes that a previous venipuncture site is tender and erythematous with a red streak extending 4 inches above the site, the likely cause is _____.

    a. allergic response
    b. hematoma
    c. ecchymosis
    d. phlebitis

111. Blood draws for a GTT are usually done at _____.

    a. 30 minutes, 1 hour, 2 hours, and 4 hours
    b. 30 minutes, 60 minutes, 90 minutes, and 2 hours
    c. 2 hours, 4 hours, 6 hours, and 8 hours
    d. 1 hour, 2 hours, and 3 hours

112. Separated serum or plasma specimens should be maintained at room temperature for no more than _____.

    a. 2 hours
    b. 4 hours
    c. 6 hours
    d. 8 hours

113. Which of the following should NOT result in a lawsuit for negligence?

    a. Doing a fingerstick on a 6-month-old infant
    b. Providing information about a test to a child's mother
    c. Misidentifying a patient
    d. Lowering a bedrail and leaving it down

114. The first step in transferring blood drawn from a collecting syringe to a collecting tube is to _____.

    a. remove the needle and discard
    b. apply a blood transfer device
    c. attach a collection tube
    d. activate the needle safety features

115. The primary reason that specimens are rejected in the lab is because of _____.

   a. Breakage
   b. Overfilling
   c. Incorrect additive
   d. Hemolysis

116. If an accidental arterial puncture is suspected, the correct response is to _____.

   a. complete the draw and apply immediate pressure to the site
   b. withdraw the needle immediately and apply pressure to the site
   c. complete the draw and observe the puncture site for edema, bleeding
   d. leave the needle in place and call for help

117. Laboratory accreditation agencies generally require that laboratories follow the standards of the _____.

   a. CMS
   b. CLSI
   c. CAP
   d. FDA

118. Which of the following is an example of an immunologic test?

   a. LD
   b. RF
   c. BUN
   d. MCH

119. If a laboratory detects a suspected outbreak of an infectious disease, such as *E. coli* infections, to which governmental agency should a report be made?

   a. CLSI.
   b. USDA.
   c. NIH.
   d. CDC.

120. For blood cultures, if using iodophors for the main disinfectant, how long does it take for the iodophors to adequately disinfect the skin?

   a. 15-30 seconds.
   b. 30-60 seconds.
   c. 60-90 seconds.
   d. 90-120 seconds.

Answer Key and Explanations for Test #2

1. B: If blood must be drawn from an arm with an IV in place, the phlebotomist should ask the nurse to turn off the IV and then wait at least 2 minutes before attempting venipuncture to decrease the dilution of the blood. The phlebotomist is not allowed to adjust or stop the flow of an IV. A tourniquet must be applied, and the venipuncture is carried out distal to the IV. The phlebotomist should record the type of fluid and medication (if applicable) in the IV. The phlebotomist must notify the nurse that the venipuncture is complete and the IV needs to be restarted.

2. D: The closure cap of the collection tube that contains sodium citrate is light blue. Sodium citrate is an anticoagulant, and the cap color is color-coded so the phlebotomist can easily identify the correct tube. The blue-capped tube is utilized when conducting anticoagulant tests (PT, PTT, TT, and coagulation factors) on plasma because the anticoagulant prevents coagulation from occurring before the specimen is processed. It's important to fill the blue-capped evacuated tubes to capacity or else the results may be inaccurate.

3. D: If the phlebotomist observes another worker placing needles and syringes into a personal bag before leaving work, the best response is to notify a supervisor as soon as possible, describing in detail the observation. Confronting another person who is doing an illegal or unethical act may precipitate a violent response. Most organizations have established protocols for dealing with theft, and the supervisor should determine whether or not the police should be called.

4. B: The preferred capillary puncture site for adults and children older than 1 year of age is the distal segment of the nondominant third or fourth finger (palmar surface). The nondominant hand tends to be less calloused than the dominant hand. The tip of the finger should be avoided, and the puncture should be made perpendicular to whorls. Capillary blood should not be obtained on the same side as a prior mastectomy without written permission of the physician.

5. B: The chain of custody for a blood specimen, such as one for drug testing, begins with the initial contact with the patient when the venipuncture is carried out. A chain of custody form or other record should be filled out, and information is entered with each specimen transfer from the initial one until the final disposition. Each person involved must be identified and must sign or initialize the form/record, and each process carried out on the sample must be described. The sample must be stored in a secured and restricted storage site.

6. D: A corrosive chemical is a health hazard as opposed to a physical hazard because contact with the chemical may result in health impairment, such as loss of tissue. Other health hazards include substances that are carcinogens (cancer), irritants (eye, skin irritation), teratogens (birth defects), sensitizers (allergic response), and toxins (severe illness, death). Hazardous materials may be ingested orally, inhaled in fumes or aerosolized substances, or absorbed through the skin, eyes, or mucous membranes.

7. A: A test request should include the following specific information about the patient:

- Name: First, middle, last
- Identification (ID)/Record number
- Gender: Male, female (typically the gender assigned at birth, but this may vary to include nonbinary or transgender)
- Date of birth

139

In addition to information about the patient, the test request should include the name of the ordering health-care provider, the tests to be performed, the collection site (if appropriate), the date the collection is to be made, and any additional instructions that are necessary.

8. B: The billing code that is used for laboratory testing for inpatients is ICD-10-PCS (procedure coding system), which is used to report and bill procedures while patients are hospitalized. Outpatient procedures, on the other hand, are billed using Current Procedural Terminology (CPT) codes. ICD-11 is the code for diagnoses (replacing ICD-10-CM), but it cannot be used for billing purposes alone, although each test that is billed must contain the appropriate ICD-11 code as well for inpatients and outpatients.

9. B: According to the Americans with Disabilities Act (ADA), to ensure accessibility to patients on crutches or in wheelchairs, at least one space next to the phlebotomy chair must have a minimum area of 30 × 48 inches. Space should be available for a wheelchair to turn 180°. There must be adequate space on either side of the phlebotomy chair for transfers to and from gurneys, wheelchairs, or stretchers, and both sides must allow access to the patient. A bariatric phlebotomy chair should be available for large patients.

10. A: If a patient is very angry and yells that the lab tests are a "waste of time," the best initial response is to stay calm and listen, allowing the patient to vent. Patients are often frustrated and frightened and in pain, and these factors may cause patients to lash out at those caring for them. Once the patient has expressed his feelings and calmed somewhat, then the phlebotomist should speak calmly, expressing empathy and using the patient's name to personalize the exchange.

11. C: A blood sample in a gray-capped evacuated collection tube should be inverted a minimum of 8 times to ensure that the additive mixes adequately with the blood specimen. The gray-capped collection tube is used for glucose testing. Additives can include potassium oxalate/sodium fluoride, sodium fluoride only, or sodium fluoride/Na_2EDTA. Because glucose levels vary with intake, patients usually fast for 8 hours prior to testing unless the order specifically indicates times, such as after meals.

12. D: If protocol for blood C&S requires skin antisepsis with alcohol (isopropyl 70%) followed by tincture of iodine (2%), but the patient is allergic to iodine, an acceptable alternate procedure is to wash the skin with soap and water and when dry to cleanse twice with alcohol, allowing the skin to air dry after each cleansing. Skin asepsis is especially important with C&S because of the risk that skin bacteria will contaminate the specimen.

13. B: Reflux of an additive, especially an anticoagulant such as EDTA, may cause adverse effects if it occurs during venipuncture, so the best method of preventing reflux is to place the arm in a downward position with the collection tube below the venipuncture site so that gravity prevents reflux. Care should also be taken to prevent back and forth movement of the tube during filling as this mixes the specimen with the anticoagulant.

14. D: The non-profit organization CLSI (Clinical and Laboratory Standards Institute) determines the order of the draw and publishes this information in the publication *Procedures for the Collection of Diagnostic Blood Specimens*, which is updated periodically to reflect changes in the healthcare industry as well as findings related to research. Hospitals and other healthcare organizations should use current order of the draw unless they have evidence-based research that supports altering this order. Some newer tubes are not listed in the order of the draw, so the manufacturer's directions regarding order should be followed.

15. A: When conducting a fingerstick glucose test, to transfer the blood from the finger to the test strip, the phlebotomist should hold the edge of the strip next to the drop of blood. The blood will wick onto the strip. For most tests, the first drop should be wiped away, and the second drop is used for testing. Before testing, controls should be run to ensure that the control solution and the control strips match. After the puncture site is cleansed with alcohol, the alcohol should be thoroughly dry before proceeding.

16. C: When asked to collect blood from a peripheral vascular access device, the phlebotomist should recognize that this procedure can only be performed if the phlebotomist has completed the required training, per facility protocol. The phlebotomist may often be asked to assist in the process of blood collection from a vascular access device by passing the appropriate tubes and advising about the volume of specimens needed and the order of the draw. The filled collection tubes are usually transported to the lab by the phlebotomist.

17. D: If a patient's test request requires a chemistry panel, a CBC, a PT, and blood typing, the order in which the specimens should be drawn is:

1. PT (light-blue stopper)
2. Chemistry panel (red or gold stopper)
3. Blood typing (pink stopper)
4. CBC (lavender/purple stopper)

18. B: With double-pointed needles, the rubber sheath that covers the shorter needle is intended to prevent leakage of blood when evacuated collection tubes are changed for multiple collections or when the final evacuated collection tube is removed. The sheath retracts when a tube is pushed onto the needle to collect a sample and then covers the needle again as the tube is removed. This transfer needle is covered by a protective tube holder, which must be left in place for disposal.

19. D: If an indwelling line, such as a central venous catheter, is used to obtain a blood sample, 5 mL of blood should be discarded before the sample of blood is collected in order to clear the sample of any intravenous fluids or medications that were administered through the central venous line. In some cases, the initial blood withdrawn is readministered to the patient after the specimen is obtained in order to prevent iatrogenic anemia.

20. D: Blood cultures cannot be carried out on a specimen obtained through heelstick because there is a potential for contamination. Coagulation studies also cannot be carried out with a capillary sample. Capillary tests can only be carried out if a small quantity of blood is necessary. Tests that can be carried out include most chemistries, CBC, blood gas analysis, toxicology tests, liver function tests, and newborn screening. Capillary collection may be used for infants as well as adults.

21. C: Using a foot vein for a blood draw increases risk of blood clots because circulation is often impaired in the legs and feet, especially with older and/or diabetic patients. Patients are also at increased risk of ulceration of the site. Drawing blood from the foot or ankle should be avoided although, if neither arm can be used, then blood may be drawn from the foot or ankle with a physician's order.

22. C: If a phlebotomist sustains a needlestick injury, the first step is to immediately wash the puncture site with soap and water. As soon as possible, the supervisor should be notified and the injury reported according to protocol. The patient source should be identified so that the person can be tested for HIV, HBV, and HCV with consent. The phlebotomist should report to the designated health service so that testing procedures can be outlined and PEP (post-exposure prophylaxis) started.

23. A: Underfilling a green-capped evacuated collection tube may result in low test results because this results in excess heparin and dilution effect. The minimal acceptable draw volume for the green-capped collection tube is 50%. Overfilling, on the other hand, may result in insufficient heparin to prevent clotting, so clots may form. If this occurs, then the blood sample must be discarded and a new specimen obtained. The green-capped tube may contain either lithium heparin or sodium heparin, and is used for chemistry test on plasma.

24. A: When doing a venipuncture for a complete blood count (CBC), the stopper color that indicates the correct tube is lavender/purple. This tube is used for CBC, differential, reticulocyte count, sedimentation (sed) rate, platelet count, Coombs test, cyclosporine test, and flow cytometry. The light-blue tube (3.2% sodium citrate) is used for coagulation tests such as PT, PTT, and thrombin clotting time. The pink tube (K2 EDTA) is used for blood typing and screening, direct Coombs, and HIV viral load. The green tube (sodium heparin 100 USP units) is used for ammonia, lactate, and human leukocyte antigen typing.

25. D: If a patient has paralysis and lack of sensation in the right arm and hand, the best choice for venipuncture is any appropriate site on the left arm. With paralysis, muscle tone is lost, and this may cause some pooling of blood, increasing the risk of thromboses. Additionally, the lack of sensation means that if a nerve is inadvertently injured, the patient will be unaware. If venipuncture from a paralyzed limb cannot be avoided, then the phlebotomist should follow procedures carefully and avoid any lateral probing and ensure that pressure is held on the puncture site until any bleeding has stopped.

26. D: For venipuncture, the vein should be anchored distal to the puncture site, safely out of reach of the tip of the needle by 1–2 inches. The thumb of the free hand is used to anchor the vein with a downward pull so that the skin is taut. The vein should not be anchored on either side or proximal to the puncture site because this increases the risk of accidental needlestick injury and may impede acquisition of the blood sample.

27. A: The greatest risk when a tube breaks during centrifugation is aerosolization of the specimen because the spinning specimen breaks down into droplets, which can be easily inhaled or can land on exposed skin, increasing risk of infection. Aerosolization can also occur if collection tubes are overfilled or if the caps come off during processing. Additionally, care must be used if removing a cap after centrifugation. Buckets, tubes, and rotors should be carefully spaced and balanced before centrifugation.

28. C: A person with blood type AB+ should receive a transfusion with blood type AB+. While blood type AB+ is considered the "universal recipient" because in an emergency, the person can receive A+, B+, AB+, or O+ blood types, other types of blood may still have antibodies (anti-A or anti-B) that may in some cases cause agglutination. If it is necessary to administer a type different than AB+, then it should be administered slowly (usually as packed cells) and the patient monitored closely.

29. B: If the phlebotomist is asked to transport a nonblood specimen, such as a urine sample, to the laboratory for testing, the phlebotomist should verify that the specimen is labeled correctly. The label should be on the container and not the lid (which must be removed for testing) and should contain the same type of identifying information as on the blood sample containers. Additionally, the type and source of the sample should be identified on the label because different types of samples may have similar appearances.

30. B: A vital function of the capillaries is to exchange gases (carbon dioxide [CO_2] for oxygen), nutrients, and metabolic by-products (wastes). Capillaries are extensions of arteriole endothelium and are tiny, thin-walled vessels that carry a mixture of arterial and venous blood. The walls of the capillaries are semipermeable with tiny openings where endothelial cells in the walls overlap. The density of capillary networks depends on the metabolism of the tissue, so capillaries are dense in muscle and nerve tissue and are less dense in cartilage, the epidermis, and the corneas.

31. D: If the phlebotomist is accidently splashed with a highly toxic hazardous chemical, the minimum length of time that the affected body part should be flushed with water is 15 minutes. The phlebotomist should know the locations of safety showers as well as eye wash stations and should immediately follow procedures for decontamination. Once the phlebotomist completes the shower or flushing of the affected body part, the person should immediately go to the health services, such as the emergency department, for evaluation.

32. A: When reviewing orders, the abbreviation for the thyroid hormone triiodothyronine is T_3, which is the active form of thyroxine. The T_3 level increases with hyperthyroidism and decreases with hypothyroidism. T_4 is the abbreviation for thyroxine; TSH, for thyroid stimulating hormone; and TBG, for thyroxine-binding globulin. Orders for tests with similar abbreviations should always be double-checked to ensure that the correct blood sample is obtained and the correct test is conducted.

33. C: When collecting a blood specimen in a collection tube that contains an additive, the collection tube should be lower than the puncture site to ensure that the additive does not come in contact with the needle because this can result in reflux of the additive into the patient's vein. The collection tube should fill from the bottom up, and movement that causes the blood to move about in the tube should be avoided. If blood is being withdrawn slowly and there is concern that clotting may occur, the collection tube should be removed, inverted for mixing, and quickly replaced into the holder.

34. D: The primary use of non-additive evacuated plastic collection tubes is for discard tubes when a few mL of blood must be discarded prior to collection of the sample. If, for example, a winged infusion set ("butterfly") is used to draw a blood sample, which is to be collected in a light blue (citrate) capped evacuated tube, then a discard tube must be used first to ensure that all dead space in the needle and tubing is filled with blood before the sample is collected to make sure the ratio of blood to additive is correct.

35. A: The Clinical and Laboratory Standards Institute (CLSI) provides standards for a wide range of performance and testing and covers all types of laboratory functions and microbiology. The institute comprises representatives from the profession, industry, and government. These standards are used as a basis for quality control procedures. Standards include labeling, security/information technology, toxicology/drug testing, statistical quality control, and performance standards for various types of antimicrobial susceptibility testing.

36. B: The left atrioventricular valve of the heart is called the mitral valve. After the blood flows into the right atrium, it flows through the tricuspid valve to the right ventricle; from there it travels through the pulmonic valve to the pulmonary arteries and to the lungs for oxygenation. The blood returns through the pulmonic veins into the left atrium and then through the mitral valve to the left ventricle and out the aortic valve to the general circulation via the aorta.

37. D: The Joint Commission is primarily an accrediting organization, accrediting healthcare facilities and programs nationally and internationally. The Joint Commission accredits hospitals, critical access hospitals, ambulatory care centers, behavioral healthcare programs, home care (plus pharmacy), laboratories (hospital-based and free standing), and nursing care centers. The Joint

143

Commission also offers a number of certificates (palliative care, disease-specific care, staffing, integrated care, and primary care medical home), indicating that a program has met specific standards.

38. D: When delivering a blood specimen that requires STAT (immediate) testing to the laboratory, the phlebotomist must notify the testing personnel and receive verbal acknowledgement of a STAT specimen. Even if a STAT rack is available, simply placing the specimen in the rack is not sufficient because personnel who are busily engaged in testing may not notice that a specimen has been placed in the rack, resulting in delays in getting the test results.

39. C: If petechiae are noted on the patient's skin distal to the tourniquet, this suggests that the patient may have a coagulation defect, such as thrombocytopenia, and may have excessive bleeding after venipuncture. Other causes of petechiae can include medications (aspirin, anticoagulants) and some types of infectious/inflammatory disorders. Petechiae are nonraised lesions that are small (<3 mm) in diameter.

40. B: The correct method of removing a stopper from a specimen tube is to pull it straight up and away from the tube. If possible, a removal device or robotics should be used to minimize human contact. Any fluid in contact with the stopper may become aerosolized when the stopper is removed; therefore, if a tube does not have a built-in safety feature to prevent aerosolization, then the stopper should be grasped with a gauze pad or a tissue.

41. D: The government agency responsible for laws governing the use of gloves when carrying out a venipuncture is OSHA under the Bloodborne Pathogen standards, with the current version part of the Needlestick Safety and Prevention Act (2000). This Act was enacted to reduce the risk of needlestick injuries and blood contamination by healthcare workers and has promoted the use of safer medical devices and work practices. States may have their own OSHA-approved programs but must meet the minimum standards developed by OSHA.

42. B: Iatrogenic (treatment-caused) anemia in a neonate is caused by excessive blood draws and is the primary reason that neonates in the NICU (neonatal intensive care unit) require transfusions. Life-threatening loss of blood occurs with loss of 10% of the total volume at one time or over a short period of time. Blood draws should be done very carefully on neonates, obtaining the minimum blood needed, making sure that draws are within established guidelines for the infant's weight.

43. A: For therapeutic drug monitoring, critical times include the time of the last dose and the time that the specimen was collected. The times should be carefully recorded to ensure that the peak level or trough level is accurately assessed. Peak levels are drawn at the time that the medication's concentration in the blood should be highest. Trough levels are usually drawn immediately before the next dose when the concentration is the lowest. The last dosage administered and the mode of administration must also be recorded.

44. B: Physician office laboratories are most often accredited by COLA (Commission on Laboratory Accreditation), founded in 1988 with the original intent of inspecting and accrediting physician office laboratories to ensure that they were in compliance with CLIA (Clinical Laboratory Improvement Amendments). COLA has since expanded its mission and now also accredits hospital laboratories as well as independent laboratories. CMS (Centers for Medicare and Medicaid Services) and the Joint Commission have granted deeming authority to COLA.

45. A: When using an evacuated tube system for venipuncture, the phlebotomist can determine that a tube is properly filled when the vacuum is exhausted. Each different type of tube has a vacuum that will provide the volume necessary for the type of test. For example, the volume of the light-blue tube is 4.5 mL, but the volume of the gold-top serum separator tube is 6 mL. Volumes typically range from 2.0-8.5 mL. The tube should also be examined after filling to ensure that it appears to contain the correct volume.

46. B: When using micro-collection tubes for a finger stick, the collection tube that should usually be filled first is the lavender-capped tube (different from the order used with venipuncture) to ensure that the volume collected is sufficient for hematology tests. This is followed by other collection tubes that contain additives, and the plain tubes utilized for serum collection are filled last. In most cases, the first drop of blood is wiped away and the second drop of blood is collected.

47. B: The governmental agency that requires an exposure control plan that outlines methods to reduce staff injury and exposure is the Occupational Safety and Health Administration (OSHA). OSHA requires that the working environment and working conditions be safe and free of recognized dangers. OSHA also requires that hepatitis B vaccines be available to all health-care workers. OSHA develops and enforces standards of workplace safety and health. Workers may file a complaint with OSHA if the workplace is out of compliance.

48. C: The correct collection tube for ethanol level (blood alcohol level) is the gray-capped tube that contains the antiglycolytic agent sodium fluoride. Antiglycolytics are agents that prevent glucose (blood sugar) from breaking down, so the gray-capped collection tube is used to check glucose levels (FBS). Because glycolysis can break down ethanol and decrease ethanol levels, the specimen must be collected in a collection tube with an antiglycolytic.

49. B: The primary function of WBCs (white blood cells/leukocytes) is to fight infection. There are 5 types of WBCs in circulation. Granulocytes are WBCs with granular cytoplasm, while agranulocytes lack these granules. Granulocytes are about two times bigger than RBCs and include neutrophils, eosinophils, and basophils. These cells develop in the red bone marrow but live only about 12 days. Agranulocytes include monocytes and lymphocytes, also formed in the red marrow. Monocytes live for weeks to months while lymphocytes may live for years.

50. A: Removing the stoppers from blood specimen tubes during the precentrifugation period can result in an increase—not a decrease—of pH because of a loss of carbon dioxide (CO_2). Other problems that may occur if a stopper is removed is evaporation of the specimen, resulting in concentration, which can alter the test results. An opened specimen container also always runs the risk of contamination. Containers should be maintained in an upright position with the stoppers in place.

51. D: Blood must be drawn from an artery for blood gases. Because arteries tend to be deeper, have thicker walls, and be in closer proximity to nerves, withdrawing blood from arteries is more difficult than from veins and must be done by someone trained to do the procedure, such as an RN, when it is within the person's scope of practice. Additionally, arterial blood draws, usually done in the wrist, are more painful than venous blood draws and may result in bleeding, hematoma, ecchymosis, and infection.

52. D: The innermost layer of an artery is the endothelium. Arteries have three distinct layers. The endothelium is normally smooth to facilitate flow of blood and it secretes biochemicals that prevent platelet aggregation (clumping). The next (middle) layer, the tunica media, is the thickest because it comprises smooth muscle and connective tissue that provide elasticity so that the artery can maintain pressure but accommodate extra blood flow when the ventricles contract. The outer layer, the tunica externa (adventitia) is thin and is connective tissue that attaches the artery to tissues.

53. A: When using a pediatric vein transilluminator with an infant, the transilluminator should be placed in the palm of the child's hand. The light projects through the hand and helps the phlebotomist locate the veins in the hand. Adult transilluminators are held onto the skin and project light downward to help illuminate the veins. The adult device has a horseshoe shape, so it can illuminate the veins from three sides. Transilluminators require a second person to hold the device in place during the venipuncture.

54. C: When loading a centrifuge that holds multiple tubes, if only one tube needs to be centrifuged, the phlebotomist should place the tube and a tube filled with the same volume of water across from it in the centrifuge. The centrifuge must be balanced: The tubes are filled with an equal volume opposite each other to prevent vibration that may result in tubes being broken and samples aerosolized. If vibration occurs after the centrifuge is turned on, this often indicates an unbalanced load and requires that the centrifuge be immediately turned off.

55. A: The blood specimen for cold agglutinins must be maintained at body temperature through warming. Another test that requires the specimens to be warmed is cryoglobulin. Usually, the specimen is collected into tubes that are pre-warmed and then placed within one minute into a temperature-controlled environment, such as an insulated container with a water bath. The temperature should be maintained at 37 °C until the specimen is processed. Laboratory guidelines should always be assessed for proper transport of specimens.

56. B: The vein-finder device that projects a pattern map of the veins on the skin is the near-infrared light device. The device is held above the skin, and the veins are outlined on the skin surface as the veins absorb the infrared light while the infrared light is reflected off of the other tissue. Infrared vein finders are available in mounted (for hands-free use) or handheld versions. The devices are especially useful with patients who have poorly visible veins and/or dark skin.

57. B: OSHA requires that employers provide healthcare workers with the appropriate PPE (personal protective equipment) at no cost in order that they can perform their job functions safely without risk of infection or injury. PPE equipment may vary according to the job description, but should include gloves, masks, face shields, shoe coverings, hair coverings, and protective gowns as well as N-95 respirators, as indicated. Additional PPE are required for those caring for Ebola patients.

58. D: When using an evacuated tube system for venipuncture, the phlebotomist must rely on sensing a decrease in resistance to determine if the needle is correctly positioned in the vein. There is no flash of blood with an evacuated tube system, only with a needle and syringe. If the phlebotomist notes that the needle is vibrating, this is an indication that the needle is in a valve and needs to be repositioned. No blood will flow into the holder until the vacuum tube is inserted.

59. A: If a coagulation test requires platelet-poor plasma, it is necessary to centrifuge the specimen, carefully remove three-quarters of the plasma at the surface (avoid pouring), place it into an aliquot tube, and then centrifuge the aliquot tube to separate any remaining cells. Then, the plasma from the second centrifugation is transferred via a new pipette into another new tube for testing. Because platelets contain clotting factors, it is essential to remove platelets before carrying out the tests. Platelet-poor plasma should have fewer than 10,000 platelets/μL.

60. C: When transporting a specimen at room temperature, an appropriate temperature is 22° C (71.6 °F). Specimens that are transported or handled at room temperature should be maintained in an environment that ranges from 20 °C to 30 °C (68 °F to 86 °C), although some measurands may begin to deteriorate with extended temperatures greater than 22 °C (71.6 °F). Specimens that must be maintained at body temperature should be kept at 36.4 °C–37.6 °C (96.8 °F–99.7 °F). Specimens transported and handled in the wrong temperature range may be altered.

61. D: When opening and aliquoting a specimen, the required PPE includes gown, gloves, and face shield. Otherwise, the opening must occur behind a portable splash screen that is placed between the specimen and the person's body. The sample should be removed from the tube with a disposable pipette and placed into the aliquot tube. Pouring the specimen from the specimen tube into the aliquot tube must be avoided because this may result in aerosolization.

62. B: When collecting blood samples in evacuated collection tubes that contain sodium citrate or ACD (acid citrate dextrose), the ratio of blood to additive must be 9:1 (draw to the 10 mL marking). Sodium citrate and ACD are both anticoagulants that stop blood clotting in the collection tube. Maintaining the proper ratio is important to ensure that the anticoagulant has the correct effect. Sodium citrate is in blue-capped tubes and ACD in yellow-capped tubes.

63. B: The phlebotomist should evaluate the risk of violence with all patients. While some patients may show outward signs of impending violence, such as by making threatening gestures or using abusive language, others (such as patients with dementia) may seem outwardly calm but react violently to venipuncture. If the phlebotomist fears violence, the phlebotomist should make sure that the exit is clear and that another staff person is in attendance to help if necessary. The phlebotomist should remain calm and speak in a soothing manner.

64. D: If an elderly patient has rolling veins, the best solution is to anchor the vein with the thumb directly distal to the puncture site, applying slight downward pressure to stretch and hold the vein in place. Rolling veins are common in elderly adults of both genders because the supportive tissue is weaker and fails to secure the vein. The arm should be extended as much as possible if using the antecubital space for the venipuncture.

65. C: For venipuncture, the vein that should always be selected as the last option is the basilic vein because it lies near the brachial artery, so accidental arterial puncture may occur. Additionally, nerves run parallel to the basilic vein, increasing the risk of injury to the nerve. The order of veins is median cubital, cephalic, basilic, dorsal metacarpal, and wrist. This means that the veins should be inspected in this order, but for venipuncture, the basilic vein goes to the end of the list.

66. A: Bloodstained gauze should be disposed of in a biohazard waste container but not in a sharps container. All used needles and lancets should be placed in the sharps container. Any sharp should also be placed in the sharps container if the package is opened, even if the sharp is unused, because the purpose of the sharps container is to prevent both transmission of disease as well as trauma. Sharps containers are often red in color.

67. D: Metal filings ("fleas") may be used with capillary blood gas collection tubes to mix blood with the anticoagulant in the tube. They are inserted into the tube and serve as stirrers. The capillary blood gas collection tubes are long and thin and commonly hold up to 100 mcL of blood. A band around the tube identifies the additive, most commonly a green band indicating the additive sodium heparin. A magnet may also be used to mix the specimen. The magnet fits over the tube and is slid up and down the length of the tube.

68. D: If a very small hematoma is evident during venipuncture, the best initial response is to observe the site and complete the venipuncture. If, however, the hematoma is large or expanding, then the phlebotomist should remove the needle, elevate the arm above the level of the heart, and apply pressure until the bleeding stops. Small hematomas are fairly common, especially in those taking anticoagulants and certain other drugs, as well as older adults, whose veins may be friable.

69. A: Steps that can help prevent the development of a hematoma include:

- Maintaining the position of the needle throughout the specimen collection
- Removing the tourniquet before removing the needle
- Removing the tube from the holder before removing the needle
- Examining the puncture site to ensure it is properly sealed prior to applying a bandage

If bruising, swelling, or other signs of a hematoma are evident during collection, the needle must be removed immediately and pressure must be applied to the site.

70. D: If a gray-capped collection tube, which is used for glucose testing, is overfilled, the result may be clotting of the specimen because overfilling results in an inadequate amount of additive needed to inactivate clotting. Therefore, the specimen must be discarded. Underfilling a gray-capped collection tube, on the other hand, causes a dilution effect and the excess additive may result in low test results. The minimum draw volume is 50% of capacity.

71. B: Sputum specimens should ideally be obtained first thing in the morning upon arising because patients tend to cough up secretions that have pooled during the night, so it is easier to get a large volume of sputum. Sputum should be obtained at least 1 hour after eating so it is not contaminated with food particles or vomitus. Before obtaining the specimen, the patient should be asked to remove dentures and to thoroughly rinse the mouth with water and gargle to reduce contaminants.

72. D: Alcohol-based antisepsis is more commonly used than povidone-iodine–based antisepsis because povidone-iodine is more likely to cause allergic response; many people are allergic to iodine. In most cases, the antiseptic of choice is 70% isopropyl alcohol in individually wrapped containers. Povidone-iodine has long been used for blood cultures and blood gases because it provides strong antisepsis, but its use is becoming less common. Other antiseptics include benzalkonium chloride, chlorhexidine gluconate, and hydrogen peroxide.

73. C: After birth, RBCs (red blood cells) are produced almost exclusively in the red bone marrow. RBCs enter the bloodstream as reticulocytes and mature into erythrocytes as the reticulum (netlike structure) degenerates. Production of RBCs increases in response to oxygen deficiency. The production of RBCs is controlled by erythropoietin, primarily released from the kidneys (and to a lesser degree by the liver). As oxygen levels improve, release of erythropoietin decreases, causing RBC production to decrease.

74. B: During venipuncture, if the needle appears to be in the vein but no blood is flowing and a slight vibration or quiver of the needle is noted, the most appropriate initial response is to remove the vacuum tube, pull back slightly on the needle, and reinsert the vacuum tube. If this is not successful, the venipuncture should be discontinued and another site is tried. The lack of blood flow and vibration/quiver suggest that the needle is in a valve, and the valve is attempting to open and close.

75. C: For the C-urea breath test, used to detect *Helicobacter pylori* infection (a common cause of stomach and duodenal ulcers), the patient exhales into a Mylar balloon for a baseline breath sample and then drinks a solution containing synthetic urea, which contains carbon 13. A second exhalation sample is then obtained 15 minutes after the patient ingests the solution. If *H. pylori* is present, it will metabolize the synthetic urea and release CO_2 containing the carbon 13, which can be detected in the breath sample.

76. A: If serum appears milky, this likely indicates lipemia, which is an increase in lipids (fats) from ingestion of foods high in fat, such as bacon, or from some intravenous feeding solutions. Lipemia

148

may be evident for up to 12 hours after ingestion, so when tests on lipids, such as triglycerides, are done, people are asked to fast for 12 hours before the test. Additionally, if the serum is lipemic, it may interfere with some chemistry tests.

77. A: An electrolyte panel includes CO_2 (carbon dioxide), Cl (chloride), K (potassium), and Na (sodium). Tests can be done using either plasma or serum. Evacuated collection tubes that can be used for the electrolyte panel include red-capped, red/black-capped SST, and green top. If the collection tube contains a clot activator, it should be inverted a minimum of 5 times. If the collection tube contains lithium heparin, an anticoagulant, it should be inverted at least 8 times.

78. B: Within a 24-hour period for pediatric or critically ill patients, the percentage of total blood volume that can be collected is 1–5% up to a total of 10% over an 8-week period. Therefore, it is important to estimate the total blood volume and to monitor the volume of blood withdrawn in order to prevent iatrogenic anemia and/or hypovolemia. In some cases, it may be advisable to obtain capillary blood for tests to decrease the volume of blood needed, especially for young children.

79. C: After using a needle and tube holder to collect a blood specimen, the tube holder should be disposed of as one unit with the needle in the sharps container. Removing the tube holder is prohibited by OSHA because doing so increases the risk of needlestick injuries. Additionally, the tube holder may be contaminated with small particles of blood and cannot be reused or resterilized but must be disposed of after use.

80. A: The purpose of a Vein Entry Indicator Device (VEID) is to indicate when a needle penetrates a vein in order to increase the success rate for venipuncture, especially in individuals with small, fragile veins, those with excessive blood loss, and those with hard-to-locate veins. The needle is attached to a pressure-sensing device that notes the change in pressure when the needle penetrates a vein and emits a beep within a tenth of a second.

81. A: The tests that are typically available on a POC arterial blood gas (ABG) analyzer include the following:

- pH: Assess acidity/alkalinity
- TCO_2: Total carbon dioxide, including intermediate forms
- PO_2: Partial pressure of dissolved oxygen in the blood
- PCO_2: Partial pressure of dissolved carbon dioxide in the blood
- SO_2: Percentage of hemoglobin-binding sites occupied by oxygen in the blood
- HCO_3: Concentration of hydrogen carbonate (a by-product of metabolism) in the blood
- Base excess/deficit: Excess with metabolic alkalosis and deficit with metabolic acidosis

82. B: Asking a nurse or anyone to temporarily store a forensic specimen may violate the chain of custody. The phlebotomist obtaining the specimen should verify identification of the patient and clearly label the specimen, and should sign the chain of custody form and place the specimen into a special transfer bag that is sealed, dated, and signed by the phlebotomist to ensure that the specimen has not been tampered with in any way.

83. B: The four stages of hemostasis:

1. Vasoconstriction: Trauma to the vessel results in vasoconstriction in order to decrease loss of blood.
2. Formation of platelet plug: Platelets begin to aggregate (stick to each other) and adhere to the traumatized area, forming a plug to prevent blood loss.
3. Formation of fibrin clot: Coagulation factors create a fibrin net to capture blood cells and platelets, sealing the traumatized vessel.
4. Fibrinolysis: The clot dissolves as healing occurs.

84. B: If a patient is chewing gum when the phlebotomist arrives to collect a blood specimen, the phlebotomist should ask the patient to remove the gum before proceeding. The patient should not be eating or drinking anything or have anything in the mouth, except for what is needed for medical treatment. Because patients sometimes jerk or even faint during venipuncture, they may choke on the gum or other substance or swallow it inadvertently.

85. C: When carrying out POC testing for PT/INR with an analyzer, such as the CoaguCheck XS Plus, a capillary blood drop should generally be applied to the test strip or other collection device within 15 seconds. A capillary tube may be used to collect the drop of blood and apply it to the test strip. The drop should be transferred by holding it near the test strip or collection device while avoiding touching or wiping the blood onto the strip or device.

86. D: Most of the blood (60–70%) in the body is found in the veins, which serve as a blood reservoir. Only 10–12% is in the arteries, 4–5% in the capillaries, 10–12% in the lungs, and 8–11% in the heart. The walls of the veins have three layers, similar to arteries, but the middle muscle layer is thinner and less elastic. The lumen of the veins is typically greater in diameter than in similar arteries, allowing them to accommodate more blood flow.

87. B: If blood cannot be obtained from either arm, before a foot or ankle can be used for drawing blood, the phlebotomist should obtain a physician's order. Because circulation in the lower extremities is often impaired, using foot or ankle veins for blood specimens increases the risk of tissue necrosis, blood clots, and infection. If venipuncture in the foot or ankle is necessary, then the phlebotomist should use a 22- or 23-gauge needle and a syringe rather than an evacuated collection tube to avoid causing the veins to collapse.

88. B: Blood pressure cuffs require intermediate to low level disinfection, usually through wiping with a liquid disinfectant. While disinfection should destroy most (but not all) bacteria, viruses, and fungi, it does not destroy bacterial spores. Surgical instruments require sterilization, which destroys all microorganisms as well as bacterial spores. Cleaning, on the other hand, is all that is generally needed for windows and furniture in a waiting area where people who are clothed have sat.

89. A: The primary purpose of therapeutic drug monitoring (TDM) is to identify optimal dosing by monitoring blood levels of the drug at different time periods. Testing is often done when the medication peaks (highest blood level), which is usually 1-2 hours after oral medication, 1 hour after IM medication, and 30 minutes after IV. Testing is also done at the trough (lowest) level, which is usually about 15 minutes prior to the next scheduled dose.

90. A: If asked to draw blood from a hospitalized patient who has lost her armband, the first action should be to ask staff to replace the armband. The phlebotomist should not draw blood on any hospitalized patient unless an armband is present. Patients in the emergency department should be assigned a temporary unique identifier (such as a patient number). Outpatients do not require armbands but the phlebotomist should verify that the patient's name and birthdate or other identifying information matches that on the laboratory request forms.

91. C: The evacuated collection tube that cannot be used to collect a specimen for a BMP is the lavender-capped collection tube, which contains anticoagulant (Na_2EDTA) and is used to collect a whole blood sample for the CBC or components. Red-capped collection tubes with clot activator, red/black SST, and green-capped tubes can all be used. The BMP includes the tests on the electrolyte panel as well as the BUN, Ca (calcium), creatinine, and glucose.

92. B: If venipuncture is required for an elderly patient with obvious tremors of the upper extremities, the best solution is to ask a nurse to assist in stabilizing the arm. Equipment should be chosen carefully to avoid unnecessary trauma and prolonged venipuncture. Older adults, especially with small friable veins, may bruise easily. Coban or other nonadhesive elastic bandaging may be more appropriate than adhesive bandages because of the thinness of skin in older adults.

93. C: When carrying out a heelstick blood collection on a newborn, the maximum depth of the puncture should be equal to or less than 2 mm. In a newborn, the blood supply is typically located 0.35–1.6 mm below the skin. Thus, a 2 mm depth provides an adequate flow of blood but is generally too shallow to cause injury to the calcaneus. The heelstick should be done on the lateral aspects of the heel rather than the middle or posterior aspects to ensure that the calcaneus is avoided.

94. C: If the phlebotomist drops an unused glass collection tube, causing it to break and scatter pieces of glass, the phlebotomist should guard the area to prevent anyone from being injured and call housekeeping. The glass should be removed with a brush and dustpan. Any large pieces should be picked up with forceps or tongs and never picked up by hand because this can result in lacerations. Whenever possible, plastic containers/collection tubes should be used instead of glass to minimize risk from breakage.

95. D: The hydrogen breath test is most often used to test for lactose intolerance. Typically, exhaled breath contains very little hydrogen. However, if there is a problem with the digestions of lactose or other carbohydrates (such as fructose), bacteria in the colon ferment the carbohydrates, and this produces hydrogen, which is absorbed into the systemic circulation and sent to the lungs, from where the hydrogen is exhaled. Higher than normal levels of hydrogen suggest a problem with carbohydrate metabolism.

96. A: For forensic collection of a blood sample, the specimen container must be placed and sealed inside a transfer bag. Careful documentation regarding patient identification and date and time of venipuncture is critical to establish the chain of custody. The phlebotomist signs the transfer form and the transfer bag (if signature is required) to indicate that the chain of custody has not been breached. The bag must remain sealed until it is processed by the appropriate laboratory.

97. A: If drawing a blood specimen from an adolescent, the phlebotomist should recognize that most adolescents are self-conscious and concerned about their bodies and appearance. They may become embarrassed easily, so it is important that their privacy be maintained. Some may be afraid to express their fears in an attempt to "act like an adult," while others may act belligerently to hide fears. The phlebotomist should explain the procedure completely and ask if the patient has questions.

98. B: The order in which pediatric micro-collection containers should be collected (which differs from standard vacutainers) is lavender (which contains EDTA anticoagulant), green (which contains sodium or lithium heparin), and finally red (which does not contain additives). The lavender tube is used for standard hematology tests (such as RBC, WBC counts), which are often most important, so it should be collected first to ensure that the volume collected is adequate, since obtaining adequate amounts of blood from pediatric patients can be difficult.

99. B: Before a blood specimen is collected from a newborn for routine screening, the infant should have nursed or been bottle-fed for at least 24 hours (48 is optimal) because many IEMs are related to problems with protein metabolism; therefore, the child needs to ingest protein in order for the test results to be accurate. Because some mothers and infants are discharged within 24 hours and the tests may not be completely accurate, all mothers should be advised of the importance of a repeat screening after discharge.

100. A: Cotton balls should no longer be used to apply alcohol to the skin because small particles of lint may adhere to the skin and be injected with the venipuncture. Alcohol pads and/or povidone-iodine wipes should be used for skin antisepsis. Other equipment needed for routine venipuncture includes evacuated collection tubes, tourniquet, lint-free gauze, tape or stretch nonadhesive bandages, gloves, and syringes.

101. B: While *Mycobacterium tuberculosis* is highly infectious, better treatment and early diagnosis have markedly decreased incidence, so it is rarely a cause of nosocomial infections unless a patient has been misdiagnosed. Three common pathogenic agents associated with nosocomial (health care associated) infections are *Staphylococcus aureus,* MRSA *(methicillin-resistant Staphylococcus aureus),* and *Clostridium difficile. Staphylococcus aureus* and MRSA are often associated with wound and soft tissue infections while *Clostridium difficile* results in infection of the GI system and severe diarrhea.

102. C: Venipuncture of the basilic vein, which lies on the ulnar side of the wrist, poses the greatest risk of accidental puncture of an artery because the vein lies in close proximity to the brachial artery. The median cubital vein is relatively large and less likely to roll than some other veins, so it is usually the first choice for venipuncture followed by the cephalic vein, which lies on the radial side of the wrist. The metacarpal veins are often easily visible, but should usually be avoided in older adults because of little supporting subcutaneous tissue.

103. C: According to CLSI guidelines on the venous blood specimen collection process, the first step in carrying out a venipuncture is to identify the patient. Proper identification procedure requires the use of two identifiers. In a laboratory setting, this usually involves verifying the patient's name and birthdate by asking the patient for the information rather than providing the information and asking if it is correct. In an inpatient facility, the patient should always be asked to give his or her name and birthdate if the patient is cognizant and the name band checked as well for the name and identification number. The patient is then provided information on the procedure (including the purpose) and consent is obtained. After conducting appropriate hand hygiene, the patient is then assessed for possible complications, positioned in a reclining or seated position, the site for the venipuncture is identified, and the specimen is collected.

104. B: If a patient is very thin with prominent veins that require a low needle angle for venipuncture, the best choice is probably a winged infusion ("butterfly") set with syringe because the syringe is not attached to the needle, so it does not get in the way, allowing a very low angle for venipuncture as the needle can be held almost parallel to the skin. Most venipunctures are done at about a 30-degree angle, but each patient must be evaluated individually.

105. A: In the United States, all laboratory testing, except for research, is regulated by CMS through the CLIA. CLIA is implemented through the Division of Laboratory Services and serves approximately 244,000 laboratories. Laboratories receiving reimbursement from CMS must meet CLIA standards, which ensure that laboratory testing will be accurate and procedures followed properly. The CDC partners with CMS and the Food and Drug Administration (FDA) in supporting CLIA programs.

106. C: When collecting specimens for PT (prothrombin time), aPTT (activated partial thromboplastin time), and TT (thrombin time), the correct collection tube cap color is light blue. All three tests must be done on plasma, and in all cases the collection tube must be filled to the correct volume. These three tests are often done together as screening for coagulation disorders. Normal values (may vary slightly from one laboratory to another):

- PT: 10-13 seconds
- aPTT: 25-39 seconds
- TT: <20 seconds (usually 15-19)

107. A: If a venipuncture must be done at a specific time but the phlebotomist mistakenly collects the specimen 30 minutes late, the phlebotomist should report the late collection immediately because, depending on the type of test, the late collection may alter the results. If the situation is immediately brought to the attention of the laboratory supervisor, the specimen may be salvaged. It is unethical to fail to report an error or to hope that no one finds out.

108. C: When collecting a capillary blood specimen for bilirubin from a newborn receiving phototherapy for jaundice, it is especially important to turn off the phototherapy light during collection because exposure of the blood sample to the light may break down the bilirubin. The specimen must be obtained carefully to prevent hemolysis and placed in an amber microcollection container, or the container should be covered with aluminum foil to protect the contents from light. The blood specimen should be collected as soon after the request as possible because accurate timing can help to determine the rate of bilirubin increase.

109. C: Plasma comprises 55% of the blood volume, and 45% is other formed elements, such as white blood cells and RBCs. Plasma is the fluid portion of the blood and is composed of 91% water and 9% solutes. Solutes include gases (oxygen, CO_2, nitrogen), minerals (electrolytes), nutrients (carbohydrates, lipids), proteins (albumin), antibodies, fibrinogen, waste products (blood urea nitrogen, creatinine, uric acid), vitamins, hormones, and drugs.

110. D: If the phlebotomist notes that a previous venipuncture site is tender and erythematous with a red streak extending 4 inches above the site, the likely cause is phlebitis, which is inflammation of the superficial veins, usually in the arms if associated with IVs or venipuncture. Phlebitis, which is associated with erythema, swelling, hardening of the vein, and tenderness, is usually not infective and often resolves with application of heat. However, if infection or deep vein thrombosis occurs, the symptoms spread, the patient often runs a fever, and pain may increase markedly.

111. D: Blood draws for a GTT (glucose tolerance test) are usually done at 1 hour, 2 hours, and 3 hours after the test begins. Prior to beginning the timed portion of the test, a FBS (fasting blood sugar) is done to ensure that the level is within a safe range. If so, then the glucose solution is drunk within 5 minutes and the timed period of the test begins. The patient should be advised to eat no food and only drink water during the testing period.

112. A: Separated serum or plasma specimens should be maintained at room temperature for no more than 2 hours. This maximum time limit is used because it complies with the requirements for numerous tests, such as glucose, lactate dehydrogenase, catecholamines, lactic acid, and potassium. Processing a specimen within this time frame prevents further metabolic changes, such as glycolysis, which may affect the test results.

113. B: The parent of a minor has the legal right for information about the child's tests, so providing this information should not result in a lawsuit. However, doing a fingerstick on a 6-month-old infant increases the risk of injury to the bone as only heel sticks should be done on children younger than 1 year. Misidentifying a patient could result in a lawsuit if harm comes to the patient as a result. Lowering a bedrail and leaving it down increases the risk of patient fall and injury.

114. D: The first step in transferring blood drawn from a collecting syringe to a collecting tube is to activate needle safety features while the needle is still in the arm or immediately after it is removed, depending on the manufacturer's instructions. The needle should be removed and discarded in the appropriate container and the blood transfer device attached. Then the collection tube is inserted into the blood transfer device, puncturing the cap and transferring the sample.

115. D: The primary reason that specimens are rejected in the lab is because of hemolysis. Hemolysis may alter test results or preclude testing. Hemolysis may occur if blood is drawn from an area distal to the antecubital area, if the wrong-sized needle is used, if alcohol on the skin has not dried and contaminates the specimen, if venipuncture technique is poor, if a syringe is used to withdraw blood, and if the tourniquet is left in place for longer than a minute.

116. B: If an accidental arterial puncture is suspected, the correct response is to withdraw the needle immediately and apply strong pressure for a minimum of 5 minutes, observing the site carefully for signs of swelling or bleeding. The ordering physician must be notified, and an incident report must be completed. If a specimen was already collected before an arterial puncture was suspected, the laboratory may still be able to test the arterial blood.

117. B: Laboratory accreditation agencies generally require that laboratories follow the standards of the CLSI (Clinical and Laboratory Standards Institute). CLSI, a nonprofit membership agency, publishes the *Procedures for the Collection of Diagnostic Blood Specimens by Venipuncture; Approved Standard*, which outlines the order of the draw. CLSI provides voluntary consensus standards, guidelines, and reports as well as supporting products, such as software and wall charts. CLSI is ANSI (American National Standards Institute) accredited.

118. B: RF (rheumatoid factor) is an immunologic test done to help diagnose rheumatoid arthritis, which is an autoimmune disorder. RF is an autoantibody that combines with immunoglobulin (another antibody) to cause disease. MCHC (mean corpuscular hemoglobin concentration) is a hematological test, part of the CBC. BUN is a kidney function test. LD (lactate dehydrogenase) is a chemistry test of a substance that increases with heart attack as well as chronic liver, lung, and kidney disease.

119. D: If a laboratory detects a suspected outbreak of an infectious disease, such as *E. coli* infections, the government agency to which the laboratory should make a report is the Centers for Disease Control and Prevention (CDC), which maintains the Center for Global Health (CGH), whose goal is to protect the health and safety of Americans by tracking disease and ensuring efforts to reduce disease worldwide. The CGH monitors outbreaks throughout the world, taking measures to prevent spread, and it provides technical assistance, often in conjunction with the World Health Organization.

120. D: For blood cultures, if using iodophors for the main disinfectant, it takes 90-120 seconds to adequately disinfect the skin. The usual procedure is to cleanse the skin with a 30-second friction

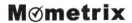

rub with 70% isopropyl alcohol, allow the alcohol to dry completely, and apply the main disinfectant and let it dry for the time recommended by the manufacturer. If the phlebotomist needs to palpate the vein after applying the disinfectant, sterile gloves must be worn.

Practice Tests #3 and #4

To take these additional practice tests, visit our bonus page:
mometrix.com/bonus948/nhaphleb

How to Overcome Test Anxiety

Just the thought of taking a test is enough to make most people a little nervous. A test is an important event that can have a long-term impact on your future, so it's important to take it seriously and it's natural to feel anxious about performing well. But just because anxiety is normal, that doesn't mean that it's helpful in test taking, or that you should simply accept it as part of your life. Anxiety can have a variety of effects. These effects can be mild, like making you feel slightly nervous, or severe, like blocking your ability to focus or remember even a simple detail.

If you experience test anxiety—whether severe or mild—it's important to know how to beat it. To discover this, first you need to understand what causes test anxiety.

Causes of Test Anxiety

While we often think of anxiety as an uncontrollable emotional state, it can actually be caused by simple, practical things. One of the most common causes of test anxiety is that a person does not feel adequately prepared for their test. This feeling can be the result of many different issues such as poor study habits or lack of organization, but the most common culprit is time management. Starting to study too late, failing to organize your study time to cover all of the material, or being distracted while you study will mean that you're not well prepared for the test. This may lead to cramming the night before, which will cause you to be physically and mentally exhausted for the test. Poor time management also contributes to feelings of stress, fear, and hopelessness as you realize you are not well prepared but don't know what to do about it.

Other times, test anxiety is not related to your preparation for the test but comes from unresolved fear. This may be a past failure on a test, or poor performance on tests in general. It may come from comparing yourself to others who seem to be performing better or from the stress of living up to expectations. Anxiety may be driven by fears of the future—how failure on this test would affect your educational and career goals. These fears are often completely irrational, but they can still negatively impact your test performance.

> **Review Video: 3 Reasons You Have Test Anxiety**
> Visit mometrix.com/academy and enter code: 428468

Elements of Test Anxiety

As mentioned earlier, test anxiety is considered to be an emotional state, but it has physical and mental components as well. Sometimes you may not even realize that you are suffering from test anxiety until you notice the physical symptoms. These can include trembling hands, rapid heartbeat, sweating, nausea, and tense muscles. Extreme anxiety may lead to fainting or vomiting. Obviously, any of these symptoms can have a negative impact on testing. It is important to recognize them as soon as they begin to occur so that you can address the problem before it damages your performance.

> **Review Video: 3 Ways to Tell You Have Test Anxiety**
> Visit mometrix.com/academy and enter code: 927847

The mental components of test anxiety include trouble focusing and inability to remember learned information. During a test, your mind is on high alert, which can help you recall information and stay focused for an extended period of time. However, anxiety interferes with your mind's natural processes, causing you to blank out, even on the questions you know well. The strain of testing during anxiety makes it difficult to stay focused, especially on a test that may take several hours. Extreme anxiety can take a huge mental toll, making it difficult not only to recall test information but even to understand the test questions or pull your thoughts together.

> **Review Video: How Test Anxiety Affects Memory**
> Visit mometrix.com/academy and enter code: 609003

Effects of Test Anxiety

Test anxiety is like a disease—if left untreated, it will get progressively worse. Anxiety leads to poor performance, and this reinforces the feelings of fear and failure, which in turn lead to poor performances on subsequent tests. It can grow from a mild nervousness to a crippling condition. If allowed to progress, test anxiety can have a big impact on your schooling, and consequently on your future.

Test anxiety can spread to other parts of your life. Anxiety on tests can become anxiety in any stressful situation, and blanking on a test can turn into panicking in a job situation. But fortunately, you don't have to let anxiety rule your testing and determine your grades. There are a number of relatively simple steps you can take to move past anxiety and function normally on a test and in the rest of life.

> **Review Video: How Test Anxiety Impacts Your Grades**
> Visit mometrix.com/academy and enter code: 939819

Physical Steps for Beating Test Anxiety

While test anxiety is a serious problem, the good news is that it can be overcome. It doesn't have to control your ability to think and remember information. While it may take time, you can begin taking steps today to beat anxiety.

Just as your first hint that you may be struggling with anxiety comes from the physical symptoms, the first step to treating it is also physical. Rest is crucial for having a clear, strong mind. If you are tired, it is much easier to give in to anxiety. But if you establish good sleep habits, your body and mind will be ready to perform optimally, without the strain of exhaustion. Additionally, sleeping well helps you to retain information better, so you're more likely to recall the answers when you see the test questions.

Getting good sleep means more than going to bed on time. It's important to allow your brain time to relax. Take study breaks from time to time so it doesn't get overworked, and don't study right before bed. Take time to rest your mind before trying to rest your body, or you may find it difficult to fall asleep.

> **Review Video: The Importance of Sleep for Your Brain**
> Visit mometrix.com/academy and enter code: 319338

Along with sleep, other aspects of physical health are important in preparing for a test. Good nutrition is vital for good brain function. Sugary foods and drinks may give a burst of energy but this burst is followed by a crash, both physically and emotionally. Instead, fuel your body with protein and vitamin-rich foods.

Also, drink plenty of water. Dehydration can lead to headaches and exhaustion, especially if your brain is already under stress from the rigors of the test. Particularly if your test is a long one, drink water during the breaks. And if possible, take an energy-boosting snack to eat between sections.

> **Review Video: How Diet Can Affect your Mood**
> Visit mometrix.com/academy and enter code: 624317

Along with sleep and diet, a third important part of physical health is exercise. Maintaining a steady workout schedule is helpful, but even taking 5-minute study breaks to walk can help get your blood pumping faster and clear your head. Exercise also releases endorphins, which contribute to a positive feeling and can help combat test anxiety.

When you nurture your physical health, you are also contributing to your mental health. If your body is healthy, your mind is much more likely to be healthy as well. So take time to rest, nourish your body with healthy food and water, and get moving as much as possible. Taking these physical steps will make you stronger and more able to take the mental steps necessary to overcome test anxiety.

Mental Steps for Beating Test Anxiety

Working on the mental side of test anxiety can be more challenging, but as with the physical side, there are clear steps you can take to overcome it. As mentioned earlier, test anxiety often stems from lack of preparation, so the obvious solution is to prepare for the test. Effective studying may be the most important weapon you have for beating test anxiety, but you can and should employ several other mental tools to combat fear.

First, boost your confidence by reminding yourself of past success—tests or projects that you aced. If you're putting as much effort into preparing for this test as you did for those, there's no reason you should expect to fail here. Work hard to prepare; then trust your preparation.

Second, surround yourself with encouraging people. It can be helpful to find a study group, but be sure that the people you're around will encourage a positive attitude. If you spend time with others who are anxious or cynical, this will only contribute to your own anxiety. Look for others who are motivated to study hard from a desire to succeed, not from a fear of failure.

Third, reward yourself. A test is physically and mentally tiring, even without anxiety, and it can be helpful to have something to look forward to. Plan an activity following the test, regardless of the outcome, such as going to a movie or getting ice cream.

When you are taking the test, if you find yourself beginning to feel anxious, remind yourself that you know the material. Visualize successfully completing the test. Then take a few deep, relaxing breaths and return to it. Work through the questions carefully but with confidence, knowing that you are capable of succeeding.

Developing a healthy mental approach to test taking will also aid in other areas of life. Test anxiety affects more than just the actual test—it can be damaging to your mental health and even contribute to depression. It's important to beat test anxiety before it becomes a problem for more than testing.

> **Review Video: <u>Test Anxiety and Depression</u>**
> Visit mometrix.com/academy and enter code: 904704

Study Strategy

Being prepared for the test is necessary to combat anxiety, but what does being prepared look like? You may study for hours on end and still not feel prepared. What you need is a strategy for test prep. The next few pages outline our recommended steps to help you plan out and conquer the challenge of preparation.

STEP 1: SCOPE OUT THE TEST

Learn everything you can about the format (multiple choice, essay, etc.) and what will be on the test. Gather any study materials, course outlines, or sample exams that may be available. Not only will this help you to prepare, but knowing what to expect can help to alleviate test anxiety.

STEP 2: MAP OUT THE MATERIAL

Look through the textbook or study guide and make note of how many chapters or sections it has. Then divide these over the time you have. For example, if a book has 15 chapters and you have five days to study, you need to cover three chapters each day. Even better, if you have the time, leave an extra day at the end for overall review after you have gone through the material in depth.

If time is limited, you may need to prioritize the material. Look through it and make note of which sections you think you already have a good grasp on, and which need review. While you are studying, skim quickly through the familiar sections and take more time on the challenging parts. Write out your plan so you don't get lost as you go. Having a written plan also helps you feel more in control of the study, so anxiety is less likely to arise from feeling overwhelmed at the amount to cover.

STEP 3: GATHER YOUR TOOLS

Decide what study method works best for you. Do you prefer to highlight in the book as you study and then go back over the highlighted portions? Or do you type out notes of the important information? Or is it helpful to make flashcards that you can carry with you? Assemble the pens, index cards, highlighters, post-it notes, and any other materials you may need so you won't be distracted by getting up to find things while you study.

If you're having a hard time retaining the information or organizing your notes, experiment with different methods. For example, try color-coding by subject with colored pens, highlighters, or post-it notes. If you learn better by hearing, try recording yourself reading your notes so you can listen while in the car, working out, or simply sitting at your desk. Ask a friend to quiz you from your flashcards, or try teaching someone the material to solidify it in your mind.

STEP 4: CREATE YOUR ENVIRONMENT

It's important to avoid distractions while you study. This includes both the obvious distractions like visitors and the subtle distractions like an uncomfortable chair (or a too-comfortable couch that makes you want to fall asleep). Set up the best study environment possible: good lighting and a comfortable work area. If background music helps you focus, you may want to turn it on, but otherwise keep the room quiet. If you are using a computer to take notes, be sure you don't have any other windows open, especially applications like social media, games, or anything else that could distract you. Silence your phone and turn off notifications. Be sure to keep water close by so you stay hydrated while you study (but avoid unhealthy drinks and snacks).

Also, take into account the best time of day to study. Are you freshest first thing in the morning? Try to set aside some time then to work through the material. Is your mind clearer in the afternoon or evening? Schedule your study session then. Another method is to study at the same time of day that you will take the test, so that your brain gets used to working on the material at that time and will be ready to focus at test time.

STEP 5: STUDY!

Once you have done all the study preparation, it's time to settle into the actual studying. Sit down, take a few moments to settle your mind so you can focus, and begin to follow your study plan. Don't give in to distractions or let yourself procrastinate. This is your time to prepare so you'll be ready to fearlessly approach the test. Make the most of the time and stay focused.

Of course, you don't want to burn out. If you study too long you may find that you're not retaining the information very well. Take regular study breaks. For example, taking five minutes out of every hour to walk briskly, breathing deeply and swinging your arms, can help your mind stay fresh.

As you get to the end of each chapter or section, it's a good idea to do a quick review. Remind yourself of what you learned and work on any difficult parts. When you feel that you've mastered the material, move on to the next part. At the end of your study session, briefly skim through your notes again.

But while review is helpful, cramming last minute is NOT. If at all possible, work ahead so that you won't need to fit all your study into the last day. Cramming overloads your brain with more information than it can process and retain, and your tired mind may struggle to recall even previously learned information when it is overwhelmed with last-minute study. Also, the urgent nature of cramming and the stress placed on your brain contribute to anxiety. You'll be more likely to go to the test feeling unprepared and having trouble thinking clearly.

So don't cram, and don't stay up late before the test, even just to review your notes at a leisurely pace. Your brain needs rest more than it needs to go over the information again. In fact, plan to finish your studies by noon or early afternoon the day before the test. Give your brain the rest of the day to relax or focus on other things, and get a good night's sleep. Then you will be fresh for the test and better able to recall what you've studied.

STEP 6: TAKE A PRACTICE TEST

Many courses offer sample tests, either online or in the study materials. This is an excellent resource to check whether you have mastered the material, as well as to prepare for the test format and environment.

Check the test format ahead of time: the number of questions, the type (multiple choice, free response, etc.), and the time limit. Then create a plan for working through them. For example, if you have 30 minutes to take a 60-question test, your limit is 30 seconds per question. Spend less time on the questions you know well so that you can take more time on the difficult ones.

If you have time to take several practice tests, take the first one open book, with no time limit. Work through the questions at your own pace and make sure you fully understand them. Gradually work up to taking a test under test conditions: sit at a desk with all study materials put away and set a timer. Pace yourself to make sure you finish the test with time to spare and go back to check your answers if you have time.

After each test, check your answers. On the questions you missed, be sure you understand why you missed them. Did you misread the question (tests can use tricky wording)? Did you forget the information? Or was it something you hadn't learned? Go back and study any shaky areas that the practice tests reveal.

Taking these tests not only helps with your grade, but also aids in combating test anxiety. If you're already used to the test conditions, you're less likely to worry about it, and working through tests until you're scoring well gives you a confidence boost. Go through the practice tests until you feel comfortable, and then you can go into the test knowing that you're ready for it.

Test Tips

On test day, you should be confident, knowing that you've prepared well and are ready to answer the questions. But aside from preparation, there are several test day strategies you can employ to maximize your performance.

First, as stated before, get a good night's sleep the night before the test (and for several nights before that, if possible). Go into the test with a fresh, alert mind rather than staying up late to study.

Try not to change too much about your normal routine on the day of the test. It's important to eat a nutritious breakfast, but if you normally don't eat breakfast at all, consider eating just a protein bar. If you're a coffee drinker, go ahead and have your normal coffee. Just make sure you time it so that the caffeine doesn't wear off right in the middle of your test. Avoid sugary beverages, and drink enough water to stay hydrated but not so much that you need a restroom break 10 minutes into the test. If your test isn't first thing in the morning, consider going for a walk or doing a light workout before the test to get your blood flowing.

Allow yourself enough time to get ready, and leave for the test with plenty of time to spare so you won't have the anxiety of scrambling to arrive in time. Another reason to be early is to select a good seat. It's helpful to sit away from doors and windows, which can be distracting. Find a good seat, get out your supplies, and settle your mind before the test begins.

When the test begins, start by going over the instructions carefully, even if you already know what to expect. Make sure you avoid any careless mistakes by following the directions.

Then begin working through the questions, pacing yourself as you've practiced. If you're not sure on an answer, don't spend too much time on it, and don't let it shake your confidence. Either skip it and come back later, or eliminate as many wrong answers as possible and guess among the remaining ones. Don't dwell on these questions as you continue—put them out of your mind and focus on what lies ahead.

Be sure to read all of the answer choices, even if you're sure the first one is the right answer. Sometimes you'll find a better one if you keep reading. But don't second-guess yourself if you do immediately know the answer. Your gut instinct is usually right. Don't let test anxiety rob you of the information you know.

If you have time at the end of the test (and if the test format allows), go back and review your answers. Be cautious about changing any, since your first instinct tends to be correct, but make sure you didn't misread any of the questions or accidentally mark the wrong answer choice. Look over any you skipped and make an educated guess.

At the end, leave the test feeling confident. You've done your best, so don't waste time worrying about your performance or wishing you could change anything. Instead, celebrate the successful

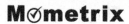

completion of this test. And finally, use this test to learn how to deal with anxiety even better next time.

> **Review Video: 5 Tips to Beat Test Anxiety**
> Visit mometrix.com/academy and enter code: 570656

Important Qualification

Not all anxiety is created equal. If your test anxiety is causing major issues in your life beyond the classroom or testing center, or if you are experiencing troubling physical symptoms related to your anxiety, it may be a sign of a serious physiological or psychological condition. If this sounds like your situation, we strongly encourage you to seek professional help.

Thank You

We at Mometrix would like to extend our heartfelt thanks to you, our friend and patron, for allowing us to play a part in your journey. It is a privilege to serve people from all walks of life who are unified in their commitment to building the best future they can for themselves.

The preparation you devote to these important testing milestones may be the most valuable educational opportunity you have for making a real difference in your life. We encourage you to put your heart into it—that feeling of succeeding, overcoming, and yes, conquering will be well worth the hours you've invested.

We want to hear your story, your struggles and your successes, and if you see any opportunities for us to improve our materials so we can help others even more effectively in the future, please share that with us as well. **The team at Mometrix would be absolutely thrilled to hear from you!** So please, send us an email (support@mometrix.com) and let's stay in touch.

> **If you'd like some additional help, check out these other resources we offer for your exam:**
> **http://MometrixFlashcards.com/Phlebotomy**

Additional Bonus Material

Due to our efforts to try to keep this book to a manageable length, we've created a link that will give you access to all of your additional bonus material:

mometrix.com/bonus948/nhaphleb

Made in the USA
Coppell, TX
22 July 2024

35005851R00096